T5-BCI-835

The Financing of Biomedical Research

The Financing of Biomedical Research

Eli Ginzberg and Anna B. Dutka

The Johns Hopkins University Press
Baltimore and London

This book is published with the generous assistance of the
Lucille P. Markey Charitable Trust.

The Johns Hopkins University Press, 701 West 40th Street, Baltimore, Maryland 21211
The Johns Hopkins Press Ltd., London

The paper used in this publication meets the minimum requirements of American National Standard for Information Sciences—Permanence of Paper for Printed Library Materials, ANSI Z39.48-1984.

Library of Congress Cataloging-in-Publication Data
Ginzberg, Eli, 1911-
The financing of biomedical research.

Includes bibliographies and index.
1. Medicine—Research—United States—Finance. 2. Medical sciences—Research—United States—Finance. 3. Medicine—Research—Finance—Government policy—United States. I. Dutka, Anna B. II. Title. [DNLM: 1. Financing, Government—trends—United States. 2. Research—United States. Q 180.U5 G492f]
R854.U5G56 1989 362.1′ 0973 88-46068
ISBN 0-8018-3813-4 (alk. paper)

Contents

Tables and Figures

Tables

Figures

Preface and Acknowledgments

This monograph was made possible by a major grant from the Lucille P. Markey Charitable Trust. It is the outcome of a suggestion made in 1984 at a meeting of the trustees and officers of the Trust and a group of consultants who had been invited to advise on the programmatic directions the trust was in the process of determining. Since the trust was directed to disburse all of its funds by 1997, the suggestion was made that a review and assessment of the financing of biomedical research would be a valuable contribution to strengthening long-term support for this important national effort.

It is hard to believe that, despite cumulative national expenditures for biomedical research of $140 billion between 1950 and 1987, few inclusive efforts have been made to trace to vast flow of resources in terms of funders and performers. The National Institutes of Health (NIH) has published the key data in comprehensive, consistent series on an annual basis, but only for the years since 1961.

We realized early on that the effort to extend the NIH data to the period before 1960 was beyond our capacity and means. Instead we concentrated on identifying and evaluating the existing information for the earlier years, which we spliced together to produce a coherent story of the flow of funds over the extended span.

Because of the special interest of the Markey Charitable Trust in the role and potential of philanthropy, particularly the roles of individual giving, bequests, and private foundations, we made a special effort to explore this little-studied sector of support for biomedical research. Chapter 6, "Academic Health Centers," is based on the replies received to a questionnaire addressed to senior administrators at ten of the nation's leading medical centers with the understanding that they would not be identified. We can therefore only make a general acknowledgment of their important contributions in responding to our questionnaire thoughtfully and promptly.

That research is a cooperative venture has been proved to us conclusively by the unstinting generosity of the many persons to whom we addressed inquiries and requests for help.

We are particularly grateful to Patricia McKinley and William Rhode of the Program Analysis Branch of the NIH, Katharine Levit of the Office of the Actuary of the Health Care Financing Administration, Betty L. Dooley, formerly of the Georgetown University Center for Health Policy Studies, Paul Jolly of the Association of American Medical Colleges and many of the staff members of the National Science Foundation and the National Science Board.

We appreciate the efforts of the American Association of Fund-Raising Counsel, Inc., publishers of *Giving USA*, and of the staffs of the Independent Sector and the Foundation Center Library, who assisted us in examining the many roles of philanthropy.

Two officials at Columbia University were particularly helpful: Patricia Francy, controller, and James Lewis, director of the Office of Projects and Grants.

We are pleased to acknowledge our debt to Harry M. Marks of the Johns Hopkins University Institute of the History of Medicine, who read the manuscript for the Johns Hopkins University Press. His review covered eleven single-spaced pages full of helpful criticisms, suggestions, and leads to sources that we had not identified. There is no question that his critique led us to improve significantly the reliability and readability of our manuscript.

Although the monograph bears the names of only two members of the staff of Conservation of Human Resources at Columbia University, it should be noted that Miriam Ostow, senior research scholar, and Howard Berliner, research scholar, participated actively at various stages of the investigation.

The successful completion of the project also benefited from the dedicated work of the support staff, particularly Sylvia Leef, Ellen Levine, and Shoshana Vasheetz.

Ruth S. Ginzberg edited the manuscript for publication, for which assistance we are duly grateful.

The Financing of Biomedical Research

1 · Overview

This study reviews and assesses one of the striking transformations in an important sector of U.S. society during the post-World War II years: the enlarged role of biomedical research on the national scene. This role has transformed the education of physicians and the practice of medicine, has contributed to the strengthening of the U.S. pharmaceutical industry, and has speeded the development of biotechnology, which, many informed observers believe, will provide a breakthrough in the economy in the decades ahead.

The single most telling piece of evidence about the changing scale of biomedical research is revealed in the total expenditures for the two years 1940 and 1987. In 1940 total outlays for biomedical research amounted to $45 million. The 1987 figure is estimated at $16.2 billion, 360 times the earlier figure.[1] In constant (inflation-adjusted) dollars, the increase is close to fortyfold.

Since ours is a pluralistic society and economy, no one sector—neither industry, nor government, nor philanthropy (nonprofit)—is solely responsible for any critical segment of the nation's output, even for defense. Just as the armed services are dependent for their weapons systems almost totally on the aerospace industry and on other parts of the civilian economy for almost all of the other goods and services they require, from food to communications, the same pattern of pluralism has characterized biomedical research. The modest research in the biomedical area that was conducted in 1940 and in the preceding decades was financed and performed by industry, the leading research universities and their medical schools, several nonprofit research institutions, and a few government agencies. Industry's funds supported more than 50 percent, universities and philanthropy slightly under 40 percent, and the federal government less than 7 percent of the total.

These figures obscure the fact that most basic biomedical research was performed then, as it is today, in research-oriented universities, in medical schools and hospitals, and in specialized nonprofit research institutions. Industry for the most part, then as now, uses its research and development (R & D) funds for applied research and development aimed at improving existing products and bringing new products to market.

The experience of the United States during World War II fundamentally altered the relationship of the key parties to the future role of research in meeting the nation's priorities. Scientists had played a leading role in assuring victory for the Allies through the development of radar and the atomic bomb. Medical scientists had played leading roles in protecting our troops from infectious diseases and, through therapeutic advances, in saving the lives of almost nineteen of every twenty battle casualties reached by a medical corpsman.

Though the outbreak of the cold war forced the federal government to look to research and development to strengthen the nation's defenses, support for science would have increased in any case since there was general agreement that science could make substantial contributions to the general welfare, including improvements in the health of the American people.

Our analysis is focused on the changing trends and patterns in the financing of biomedical research in the more than four decades since the end of World War II. By the mid-1960s the federal government had become the source of two out of every three biomedical research dollars. This new development had a major impact on universities and philanthropy, important earlier sources of the modest funds supporting basic research. The greatly increased flow of federal dollars for biomedical research, starting in the 1950s and accelerating thereafter, was directed mainly to the major research universities, which continued to be the centers where most research was conducted. Industry spent increasing amounts of its own money in its own laboratories in response to the changing market opportunities. State and local governments played minor roles either as funding agents or as performers of biomedical research.

With strong support from the White House, optimistic testimony from leading academicians that more money would enable researchers to find the causes of and cures for such dread maladies as heart disease, stroke, cancer, and other scourges, and persuasive lobbyists in Washington and the rest of the nation, Congress adopted a liberal stance toward the funding of biomedical research in the post–World War II period. This stance was maintained year after year until the federal budget came under severe pressure with the nation's increasing involvement in Vietnam in the late 1960s.

William Carey, the responsible official in the Office of the Bureau of the Budget in the early 1960s, understood that thc annual 18 percent compounded rate of increase for biomedical research (in constant federal dollars) that had occurred between 1950 and 1960 could not continue indefinitely, and he shared this observation with the leaders of academic medicine. Their initial reaction was incredulity and suspicion that Carey was unsympathetic to them and the important work on which they were engaged. It is possible, even likely, that Carey's observation was premature. If inflation had not begun to escalate with our entanglement in Vietnam, and if the new demands on the federal budget for Medicare and Medicaid (1966) had been delayed, the liberal funding trend for biomedical research might have continued for a number of years longer, but the law of compounding was certain before long to prove Carey right.

The decision to channel most of the federal dollars for biomedical research to the universities, the medical schools, and nonprofit research institutions at the end of World War II was made virtually by default. The experience of the federal government with the universities during the war had been good, and no other established institutions offered a viable alternative. American political philosophy did not favor the French and German models of government-sponsored research institutions, under ministerial direction and oversight, as the principal recipients of R & D funds.

The federal government and particularly the National Institutes of Health (NIH), the major agency with oversight over external grants for biomedical research, realized that there were serious deficiencies in the universities' infrastructures and made substantial funds available for plant, equipment, and above all, the training of research personnel. In this ongoing effort there were years, particularly between the late 1950s and the end of the 1960s, when congressional appropriations for biomedical research exceeded, in the view of informed observers, the requests for funding from capable investigators.

In this expansive environment the leading research universities, some earlier, some later, abandoned most of their caution about dependence on what was known as "soft money" and assumed that, with steadily larger flows of federal research funds, soft money, like hard money, could be used to provide tenure for many investigators. Previously, even the wealthiest universities had to add continuously to their endowments in order to expand their capital plant and recruit the additional faculty they needed to stay in the forefront. They sought to persuade large foundations, prospective individual donors, and their alumni of their need for continuing support. But with the ever-larger stream of federal dollars available to them, medical school deans and departmental chairs saw little need to continue to cultivate philanthropic sources. They increasingly concentrated their efforts on Washington.

Unfortunately, by the late 1960s and early 1970s, when the expansion of facilities and personnel had resulted in the enlargement of the research infrastructure, the flow of federal operating funds slowed considerably. The rates of increase in average annual budgetary increments that prevailed from 1950 to 1965 were reduced in the late 1960s, and, by the second half of the 1970s, Congress found it difficult to provide even a small increment in inflation-corrected dollars. In the period 1966–82, total annual federal funding for biomedical research increased by only 2.1 percent (in constant dollars) in contrast to the annual increases of 18 percent of the previous fifteen-year period (see table 2.1).

No adequate alternative source of funding was available to compensate for the decreasing rate of federal appropriations. The vastly increased role of the federal government in the financing of biomedical research had caused foundations to divert their attention to other areas. Those that continued to make sizable grants to the health area largely eschewed biomedical research but continued to support promising investigators and funded health services research. All told, philanthropy's share of total funding for biomedical research continued to decline until it stabilized at about 4 percent in the 1980s.[2]

Industry, which had previously not made significant donations to basic biomedical research conducted by universities, increased its support somewhat in the 1970s and early 1980s, but not enough to compensate for the deceleration in federal funding.

The post-1965 relative decline in federal support for biomedical research was cushioned by the expansionary stance by Congress with respect to the support of medical schools for the purpose of correcting a perceived critical shortage of physicians. In 1971 capitation payments were provided to medical and other health professional schools. This new stream of federal funds helped the academic health centers (AHCs) to adjust to the strain of constricted research dollars.

A second compensatory factor derived from the significant reimbursements the AHCs received for the care of Medicare and Medicaid patients, many of whom they had earlier treated free or for reduced charges. This created another pool of federal dollars that the vice presidents and deans of the AHCs could allocate among their combined functions of education, research, and patient care.

In 1976, after two decades of efforts by the states and the federal government to increase the number of physicians, Congress declared the physician shortage at an end. When the federal government decreased its direct financial support for medical education, the research-oriented AHCs encouraged their clinical staffs to expand or establish practice plans. This meant that many of the clinical faculty were expected to cover part or all of their salaries through consultations and patient care and that a part of the income from the practice plan, a group practice in which income is usually shared in accordance with revenue produced, would be diverted to the dean and/or the department to be used for various purposes, including the support of research.

Two further accommodations were made by the AHCs to the contraction of federal research funds. They tightened their recruitment policies and became cautious about adding staff members who could not support themselves through initial and renewed research grants. In fact, many of the departments with underfunded or unfunded members separated those who were not tenured and on occasion persuaded even tenured faculty to leave. They had more researchers than funds, but since they expected that the Congress might soon return to an expansionary stance, most of the research institutions began to undermaintain their physical facilities, using the funds "saved" to support staff.

The period between the middle of the 1970s and 1982, which included the three double-digit inflation years 1979–81, marked the nadir in federal support for biomedical research. In 1981 the level of national and federal funding in constant dollars dropped, and the decline continued in federal funding through 1982. However, as the runaway inflation was finally brought under control and as the recession of the early 1980s began to lift, the outlook brightened. The new administration of Ronald Reagan favored a shift from applied and developmental research to basic research, a policy that translated into increased funding of the major research universities.

There was a growing awareness among all leadership groups—business, labor, academia, and government—that the United States had to reassess how both its economy and its society operated if it were to become more competitive in the world economy. This growing perception of the need for reform precipitated multiple analyses of the areas of weakness and a search for ways in which the nation had begun to slip and ways in which it could recapture lost ground. Some of the answers pointed to an expanded role for science and technology, including the area of biomedical research.

In 1985 the president's science advisor asked the White House Science Council to consider the state of the major research universities and to formulate recommendations aimed at assuring their continued effectiveness in science and technology, upon which the nation's economy was increasingly dependent.

In the last few years various high-level committees have reported that the infrastructures of the research universities had been permitted to deteriorate to a dangerous level and that early remedial action was required. The deficit was estimated to be in the $10 billion range. Both a prestigious congressional committee (the House Science and Technology Committee) and a White House Science Council panel recommended that half of this required sum be covered by federal funds, the other half by state governments and philanthropy.[3]

The Congress, for its part, asked the General Accounting Office to review the strengths and weaknesses of the peer review system, which had long served as the foundation for allocating federal funds for biomedical research. Although the General Accounting Office report confirmed that there were valid objections to the peer review process, ranging from cronyism to the wasteful expenditure of talented researchers' time and effort in writing and reviewing proposals, it concluded that despite these shortcomings, peer review was considered the system of choice by seven out of eight scientists.[4]

Another problem area involves the clash between the efforts of the Office of Management and Budget to prevent escalating indirect costs from consuming an ever-increasing share of the research funds made available to federal grantees by imposing stricter regulations and the efforts of the universities to conserve the time and effort of their principal investigators for research. Some progress has recently been made on this front, but more is needed.

As a result of the new awareness that U.S. competitiveness in the international marketplace may be closely linked to the strengthening of basic research and its research-oriented universities, the director of the National Science Foundation, Erich L. Bloch, has proposed to the president the approval and funding of new science and technology centers that aim at facilitating interaction between university researchers and industry on selected frontiers, including biotechnology. The president forwarded the proposal to Congress.[5]

As the decade of the 1980s draws to a close, we find that the continued liberal funding of the major research-oriented universities has become problematic. Cross-subsidization from federal support for medical education has ended; the outlook for continuing cross-subsidization from Medicare reimbursement is bleak in light of anticipated further reductions in Medicare's funding for graduate medical education; it is unrealistic to expect much more money from faculty practice plans, which already contribute between one-third and two-fifths of medical schools' total income and are now the largest source of revenue for private medical schools. The AHCs must look once again for income from philanthropy to help them remain in the forefront of medical research. Though there is little possibility that philanthropy can replace any significant part of the federal support for biomedical research, which amounted to $7.6 billion in 1987, it can and should be encouraged to respond to two overriding challenges—to assist the major AHCs in refurbishing their infrastructures so that they will be in a better position to continue to compete for federal funding, and to finance high-risk, interdisciplinary efforts that the peer review process tends to exclude.

Fortunately, there is some evidence to suggest that philanthropic groups have begun to reassess whether they can play a constructive role in the future in the support of biomedical research, an area from which they withdrew during the earlier period of massive federal dollars. There is also considerable evidence of a much more vigorous and forceful effort on the part of the universities to tap existing and new sources of philanthropic giving that are the by-products of our dynamic economy and society.

2 · The Funding and Performance of Biomedical Research and Development

Of the total $45 million spent for biomedical research and development in 1940, the largest source of funding was industry, which spent $25 million, 55 percent of the total. Philanthropy contributed $17 million, of which $5 million represented earnings from endowments and $12 million represented grants from foundations. The federal government spent $3 million, mostly in its own laboratories.[1]

In 1987 a projected total of $16.2 billion will have been made available for biomedical research and development, a 360-fold increase, as noted, in current dollars and a 40-fold increase in constant dollars over 1940. These data reflect a greatly expanded and radically transformed set of institutional arrangements, primarily with respect to the sources of such funding (table 2.1 and fig. 2.1).

Government at all levels—federal, state, and local—is projected to provide 54 percent of the total in 1987. During the post–World War II decades, the federal government's share increased from under 7 percent of a small total in 1940 to 62 percent of a much larger total in 1965, before drifting downward to the current level of 47 percent. In 1940 the expenditures of state and local government were so small that they were not reported. In 1987 they accounted for almost $1.1 billion, or 7 percent of the total (table 2.2).

Although its relative position has never returned to the 1940 level, industry, whose share of the total had declined in the decade between 1960 and 1970 to 28 percent, once again became a major source of funds in the 1980s. In 1987, 42 percent of all funds for

Table 2.1 National and Federal Funds for Biomedical R & D, 1940–1987 (In $ Millions and Annual Compounded Rate of Increase)

	National				Federal			
	Current		Constant		Current		Constant	
	$	%	$	%	$	%	$	%
1940	45	—	155	—	3	—	10	—
1950	161	14	300	7	74	38	138	30
1955	276	11	454	9	139	13	229	11
1960	845	25	1,345	25	448	26	713	26
1965	1,884	17	2,654	15	1,174	21	1,654	18
1970	2,805	8	3,116	3	1,667	7	1,852	2
1975	4,701	11	3,811	4	2,832	11	2,259	4
1980	7,969	11	4,389	3	4,723	11	2,601	3
1981	8,645	9	4,317	−2	4,848	3	2,421	−7
1982	9,450	9	4,399	2	4,970	3	2,314	−4
1983	10,535	12	4,671	6	5,399	9	2,394	4
1984	11,899	13	5,097	9	6,087	13	2,608	9
1985	13,346	12	5,519	8	6,791	12	2,808	8
1986	14,605	9	5,790	5	6,895	2	2,733	−3
1987	16,180	11	6,156	6	7,640	11	2,907	6
1950–65				16				18
1966–82				3.2				2.1
1983–87				7.2				5.1

Source: U.S. Department of Health and Human Services, National Institutes of Health, *NIH Data Book* (Bethesda, Md., annual).

Note: Constant dollars were calculated by means of the NIH Biomedical Research and Development Price Index, 1972 = 100, from 1960 to the present. The GNP Implicit Price Deflator was used for previous years.

biomedical research and development came from this source, a share that considerably exceeded that of the NIH, although, of course, the bulk went for applied research and development, not basic research.

Total expenditures of $688 million by "private nonprofit" organizations were reported in 1987, divided in descending order among voluntary health agencies, the Howard Hughes Medical Institute, "others," and foundations. Though it increased in absolute terms over the decades, the combined total accounted for only 4.3 percent of all funds for biomedical research, a fraction of the share of 27 percent (40 percent if endowments are included) in 1940.

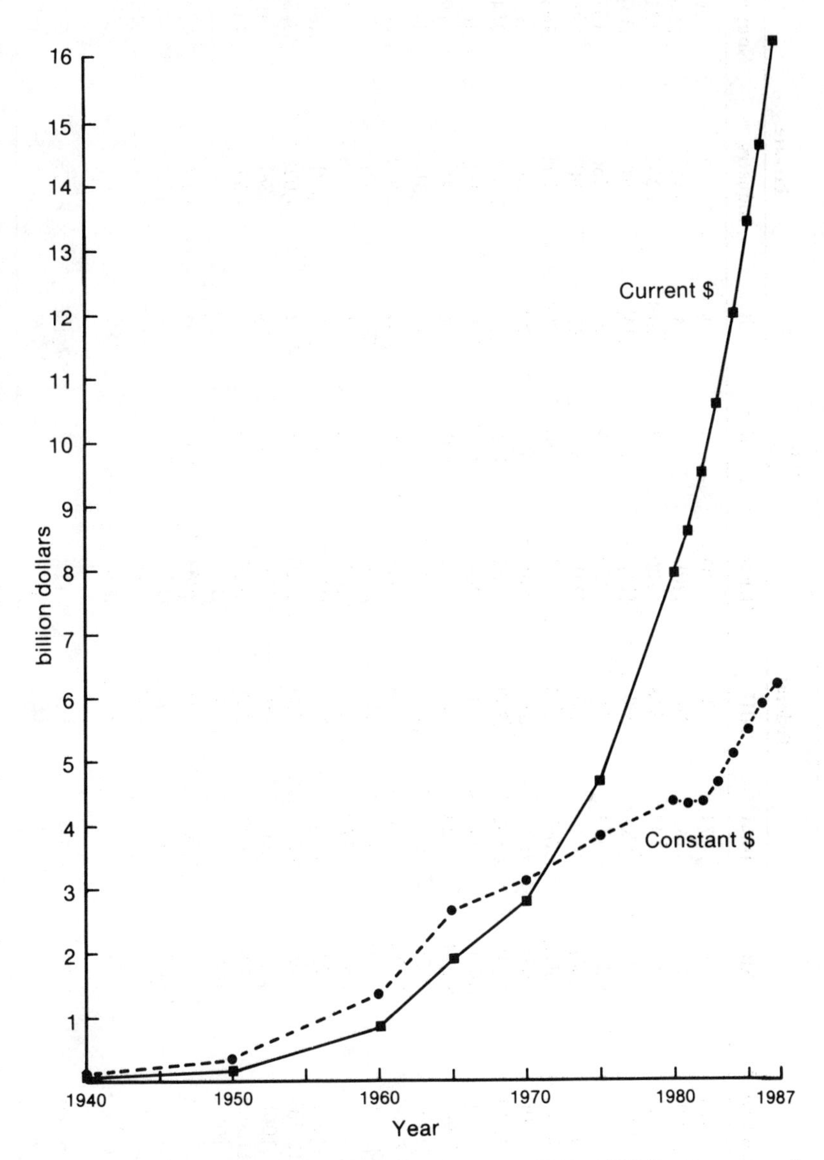

Figure 2.1 National Funds for Biomedical R & D, 1940–1987 (In Current and Constant $ Billions)
Source: Table 2.1.

Table 2.2 Sources of National Funds for Biomedical R & D, 1950–1987 (In Current $ Millions and Percentages of Total)

			Government					Private		
				Federal			State and			
		Grand Total	All	Total	NIH	Other	Local	All	Industry	Nonprofit
1950	$	161	74	74	42	32	—	87	51	36
	%	(100)	(46)	(46)	(26)	(20)	—	(54)	(32)	(22)
1960	$	845	471	448	328	120	23	374	253	121
	%	(100)	(56)	(53)	(39)	(14)	(3)	(44)	(30)	(14)
1965	$	1,884	1,277	1,174	715	459	103	607	450	157
	%	(100)	(68)	(62)	(38)	(24)	(6)	(32)	(24)	(8)
1970	$	2,805	1,817	1,667	873	794	150	988	795	193
	%	(100)	(65)	(60)	(31)	(28)	(3)	(35)	(28)	(7)
1975	$	4,701	3,118	2,832	1,880	952	286	1,583	1,319	264
	%	(100)	(66)	(60)	(40)	(20)	(6)	(34)	(28)	(6)
1980	$	7,969	5,224	4,723	3,182	1,541	501	2,769	2,466	279
	%	(100)	(65)	(59)	(40)	(19)	(6)	(35)	(31)	(4)
1981	$	8,645	5,423	4,848	3,333	1,515	575	3,200	2,921	301
	%	(100)	(64)	(57)	(39)	(18)	(7)	(37)	(34)	(3)
1982	$	9,450	5,622	4,970	3,433	1,537	652	3,712	3,504	324
	%	(100)	(61)	(54)	(37)	(17)	(7)	(40)	(37)	(3)
1983	$	10,535	6,125	5,399	3,789	1,610	726	4,410	4,035	375
	%	(100)	(58)	(51)	(36)	(15)	(7)	(42)	(38)	(4)
1984	$	11,899	6,887	6,087	4,257	1,830	800	5,012	4,525	487
	%	(100)	(58)	(51)	(36)	(15)	(7)	(42)	(38)	(4)
1985	$	13,346	7,660	6,791	4,828	1,963	869	5,686	5,190	496
	%	(100)	(57)	(51)	(36)	(15)	(7)	(43)	(39)	(4)
1986	$	14,605	7,910	6,895	5,005	1,890	1,015	6,695	5,985	710
	%	(100)	(54)	(47)	(34)	(13)	(7)	(46)	(41)	(5)
1987 (projected)	$	16,180	8,714	7,640	5,521	2,119	1,074	7,466	6,778	688
	%	(100)	(54)	(47)	(34)	(13)	(7)	(46)	(42)	(4)

Source: U.S. Department of Health and Human Services, National Institutes of Health, *NIH Data Book* (Bethesda, Md., annual).
Note: Percentage totals may not add up to 100 because of rounding.

On the performance side, the most striking finding is that, despite the very large increase in the level of funding and the substantial change in the relative positions of those who fund the research, there has been no substantial change in the positions of those who perform the research.

The Performers of Biomedical Research and Development

Between 1950 and the present the private sector has performed between three-quarters and four-fifths percent of all biomedical research (table 2.3). Whatever variability was exhibited mainly reflected changes in the role of industry as a performer and, to a far smaller degree, in the roles of government and foreign researchers. The private nonprofit sector, dominated by higher education, has consistently carried on somewhat over one-third of all biomedical research. Industry tends to perform most of the research it funds in its own facilities and, after a period of relative decline, today parallels the share of higher education. The remaining one-third is accounted for by the intramural work of federal and state government institutions and nonprofit institutions other than universities and by work done abroad with U.S. funding.

In 1987 the private nonprofit sector, primarily but not exclusively the universities and medical schools, received $6.9 billion in for biomedical research and development, 43 percent of the total. The next largest performer was industry, with outlays of $5.8 billion, 36 percent of the total. The federal government was responsible for the direct expenditure of just over $2.1 billion (13 percent), primarily for intramural research conducted in its own laboratories and, to a much lesser extent, for the management and oversight of the funds made available to its extramural grantees. State and local governments spent about $314 million in their own laboratories, accounting for only a little more than 2 percent of all biomedical research and development performed. Finally, about 7 percent ($1.06 billion) of all research and development funded by the United States was performed in foreign countries. The largest part of the overseas work was accounted for by U.S. industry, which performed 15 percent of its total biomedical research and development abroad.

In sum, the two major performers of biomedical research and development, private nonprofit institutions and industry, spent

Table 2.3 Performers of National Biomedical R & D, 1950–1987 (In Current $ Millions and Percentages of Total)

			Government			Private					
								Nonprofit			
		Grand Total	All	Federal	State and Local	All	Industry	All	Higher Education	Other	Foreign
1950	$	161	35	35	NA	126	55	71	51	NA	NA
	%	(100)	(22)	(22)	NA	(78)	(34)	(44)	(32)	NA	NA
1960	$	845	138	138	NA	707	280	427	286	NA	NA
	%	(100)	(16)	(16)	NA	(84)	(33)	(51)	(34)	NA	NA
1965	$	1,884	346	305	41	1,476	483	993	749	244	62
	%	(100)	(18)	(16)	(2)	(79)	(26)	(53)	(40)	(13)	(3)
1970	$	2,805	575	489	86	2,143	828	1,315	1,024	291	87
	%	(100)	(21)	(17)	(3)	(77)	(30)	(47)	(37)	(10)	(3)
1975	$	4,701	843	715	128	3,635	1,334	2,301	1,808	493	223
	%	(100)	(18)	(15)	(3)	(77)	(28)	(49)	(38)	(10)	(5)
1980	$	7,969	1,487	1,284	203	5,982	2,256	3,726	3,006	720	500
	%	(100)	(19)	(16)	(3)	(75)	(28)	(47)	(38)	(9)	(6)
1981	$	8,645	1,572	1,363	209	6,535	2,590	3,945	3,202	743	538
	%	(100)	(18)	(16)	(2)	(76)	(30)	(46)	(37)	(9)	(6)
1982	$	9,450	1,665	1,448	217	7,200	3,083	4,117	3,353	764	585
	%	(100)	(18)	(15)	(2)	(76)	(33)	(44)	(36)	(8)	(6)
1983	$	10,535	1,810	1,577	233	8,106	518	4,588	3,722	866	619
	%	(100)	(17)	(15)	(2)	(77)	(33)	(44)	(35)	(9)	(6)
1984	$	11,899	1,991	1,741	250	9,225	4,001	5,224	4,261	963	683
	%	(100)	(17)	(15)	(2)	(78)	(34)	(44)	(36)	(8)	(6)
1985	$	13,346	2,133	1,869	264	10,422	4,517	5,905	4,820	1,085	791
	%	(100)	(16)	(14)	(2)	(78)	(34)	(44)	(36)	(8)	(6)
1986	$	14,605	2,144	1,847	297	11,502	5,116	6,386	5,260	1,126	959
	%	(100)	(15)	(13)	(2)	(79)	(35)	(44)	(36)	(8)	(7)
1987 (projected)	$	16,180	2,417	2,103	314	12,706	5,779	6,927	5,672	1,255	1,057
	%	(100)	(15)	(13)	(2)	(79)	(36)	(43)	(35)	(8)	(7)

Source: U.S. Department of Health and Human Services, National Institutes of Health, *NIH Data Book* (Bethesda, Md., annual).
Note: Percentage totals may not add up to 100 because of rounding.

four out of every five available dollars and were followed at some distance by government (mostly federal) laboratories and foreign researchers.

When the sources of funding are juxtaposed with the performers of research, the following input-output relationships existed in 1986:

—The federal government spent 27 percent of its funds for intramural research, 73 percent for extramural. Institutions of higher education and private research organizations received almost 75 percent of all extramural funds and over one-half (53 percent) of all federal expenditures for biomedical research.
—About four out of every five dollars of state and local funds spent for biomedical research were allocated to higher education.
—Industry funded a relatively small amount of the biomedical research performed by higher education (about 4 percent) and received just over 7 percent of its total biomedical research and development funds from the federal government.
—Private nonprofit sources (philanthropy) accounted for about 11 percent of all the funds available to higher education for biomedical research.

Since industry tends both to fund and to perform most of its research and development, the interesting point of juxtaposition between funders and performers is to be found in the relationships between the principal funder, the federal government, and the principal performer, the universities, including their medical schools.

The Major Periods

Between 1950 and 1987 the average annual compounded rate of growth in biomedical research and development funds (constant dollars) came to 8.5 percent in total dollars and 8.6 percent in federal dollars.

Such averages obscure, however, the differential rates of growth that occurred over this span. There were, in fact, three distinct periods, defined by different rates of increase in funding dollars.

1. 1950–1965: rapid growth—16 percent increase in total funds, 18 percent in federal;

2. 1966–1982: slow growth—3.2 percent increase in total funds, 2.1 percent in federal;
3. 1983–1987: renewed growth—7.2 percent increase in total funds, 5 percent in federal;

These will now be analyzed in turn.

Period 1. 1950–1965: Rapid Growth

Sources of Funds

In this era of rapid growth in funding, the annual inflation rate was kept within the range of 1–2 percent, so that the difference between current dollars and constant dollars was not as large as later. A twelvefold increase in total current dollars (18 percent per year compounded) translated into a ninefold increase in constant dollars (16 percent per year compounded).

The outstanding features of this period of rapid growth were the decline in private sources of funds from 54 percent of the total in 1950 to 32 percent in 1965 and the corresponding increase in the share of public, largely federal, sources, from 46 to 68 percent (see table 2.2).

The federal government's expanded support for biomedical research and development was, as we have shown, a direct outgrowth of the nation's experience in World War II, when scientific researchers came to be viewed by President Roosevelt, the Congress, and the American people as among the architects of our victory. Vannevar Bush, President Roosevelt's senior science advisor, devoted an important part of his 1945 report, *Science: The Endless Frontier,* to the excellent prospects for achieving striking advances in the health of the American people if the government would continue and expand its funding of biomedical research.[2] Although less spectacular than the atomic bomb, radar, or sonar, important gains in medical knowledge and treatment had occurred during the war years, and it was Bush's view, based on the recommendations of his biomedical consultants, that a broadened and sustained research program could yield major gains in the future.

After the end of the war, the NIH which in 1944 had absorbed the seven-year old National Cancer Institute, was expanded to include three new institutes—Heart, Mental Health, and Dental. A number of other institutes were established later: the Eye Institute; Alcohol Abuse and Alcoholism (now combined with Mental Health in the Alcohol, Drug Abuse, and Mental Health Administration, an independent agency); Arthritis, Diabetes and Digestive and Kidney Diseases (in 1985 Arthritis was combined with Musculoskeletal and Skin Diseases in an independent institute); and Neurological and Communicative Disorders and Stroke. At present, other institutes include the National Institute on Aging, the National Institute of Allergy and Infectious Diseases, the National Institute of Dental Research, the National Institute of General Medical Sciences, the National Institute of Child Health and Human Development, and the National Institute of Environmental Health Sciences.

In the immediate post–World War II years, Congress adopted an aggressive appropriations policy for biomedical research (fig. 2.2). Its favorable stance toward the financing of medical research was strengthened because the American Medical Association had successfully lobbied against direct congressional grants for medical education, even in the face of the increasingly severe financial problems of the medical schools. Although the association opposed direct federal support of medical education because it feared Congress would seek to influence the numbers of students admitted and the curriculum, federal funds earmarked for research were considered acceptable.

It is questionable, however, even under the generally favorable economic conditions that prevailed in this period, whether Congress would have moved as energetically as it did on the R & D front—including biomedical research—had it not been for the strong and continuing encouragement that it received from several nongovernmental sectors. There was a significant number of physical scientists who had had firsthand experience during the war years with federal funding, with assembling and directing teams of co-workers, and with the advantages of ready access to large-scale support. On their return to academe, they and many of their colleagues helped to establish a favorable background for the advocates of a broadened federal commitment to biomedical research, and they received support from others who also had come to recognize the expanded potential of medicine to contribute to the general welfare. The more articulate members of this group were frequent witnesses before congressional committees.

The legislation that formally established the NIH in 1930 and

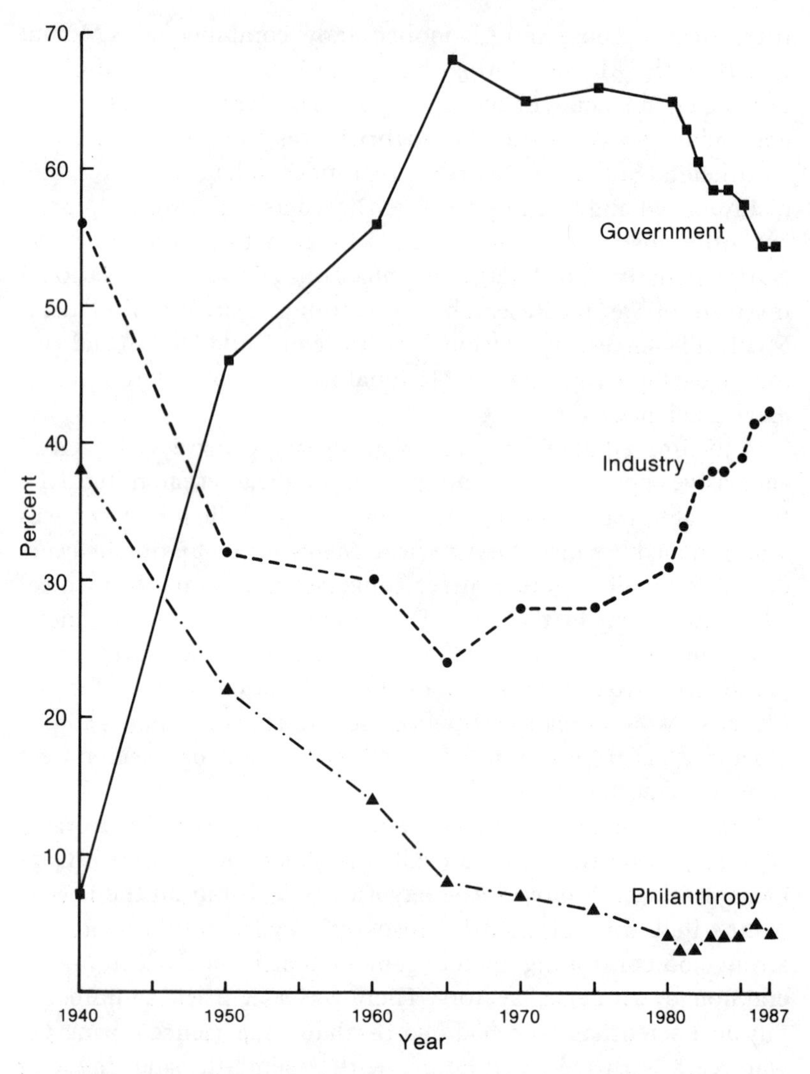

Figure 2.2 Sources of National Funds for Biomedical R & D as Percentages of Total, 1940–1987
Source: Table 2.2; 1940 data from NIH.

subsequent legislation that created successive institutes stipulated that federal funding be targeted toward disease—to find cures for diseases such as cancer, heart disease, mental illness. It was understood that the aim of federal appropriations was to increase understanding of the causes and make advances in the treatment of these and, later, still other devastating diseases. The National Science Foundation, created in 1950, had the broad mission of undertaking basic research for the purpose of enlarging the base of knowledge, but from its inception the NIH emphasized that it was seeking ways to improve the health of the American people by conquering specific diseases.

This focus on specific diseases assured that the constituencies of voluntary health agencies at national, state, and local levels would provide support when members of Congress sought to pass enabling legislation or to convince their colleagues of the need for larger appropriations. From the early days of the NIH to the present, Congress has almost always exceeded the budgetary requests for biomedical research submitted by successive administrations. A recent issue of *Science* indicates that in every year since 1970 the NIH has received more money from Congress than the president requested. Since 1933, NIH financial records reveal only eight years when the institutes did not get as much as or more than the executive branch sought.[3]

Even more than in other parts of the federal structure, close relationships developed between the chairmen of key congressional committees and the senior bureaucrats in the NIH. This made it relatively easy for the Congress during appropriations hearings to elicit unpublished information—that, for example, the requests of a particular institute for an increased budget had been turned down by the secretary of Health and Human Services, the Office of Management and Budget, or the president. And the NIH official who was testifying had little difficulty in pointing out, in answer to the committee members' questions, where and how that institute would be able to make use of additional funds.

Critically important in the formative years of the NIH were the lobbying activities of Mrs. Albert Lasker and her associates, who, convinced that research held the key to many of the nation's most devastating diseases, worked with great astuteness to convey that message to influential members of Congress, voluntary groups, and others who could help persuade Congress to appropriate ever-larger sums.[4]

But if one person is to be singled out as the principal architect of the NIH, it must be its long-term director, James Shannon, who, during his tenure between 1955 and 1968, persuaded his superiors and the key congressional leaders that the United States faced a unique opportunity to strengthen the scientific basis of modern medicine by liberal support for biomedical research, including the training of a large corps of competent investigators. This is Shannon's recent summary of his approach:

It would have been unwise in the early days of program development, 1955 through 1957, to attempt to define targets within the complexities of the many chronic diseases of concern to NIH. Rather, the immediate objectives were to increase the order of magnitude of the effort, provide a broader base of understanding of the biological systems involved, and with an increasing knowledge of the natural history of a disease, approach its solution in an opportunistic fashion. From such an approach, major lines of profitable investigation would arise. The fields of concern to NIH seemed at the time ready to burst open, and the situation would be best handled with a very loose rein.[5]

What is not immediately self-evident from this quotation is the extent to which Shannon succeeded in developing flexibility in the pursuit of biomedical research in terms of "a broader base of understanding of the biologic systems involved and with an increasing knowledge of the national history of a disease" without directly confronting the multiple external groups whose interests were focused on funding for specific diseases.

Like the federal government, industry also concluded from its wartime experience that it should initiate or expand its funding for R & D. Prior to the war, only a relatively few large U.S. corporations such as General Electric, DuPont, and AT&T (Bell Laboratories) had significant in-house R & D operations. The leading pharmaceutical companies had launched sizable R & D efforts after World War I, but they recognized the advantages of making much larger investments in biomedical research after World War II. Industry's outlays grew substantially.

Performers

In 1950 the federal government performed 22 percent of all research and development in its own laboratories, the private sector 78 percent, distributed between industry (34 percent) and the nonprofit sector (44 percent). Higher education alone was responsible for 32 percent (see table 2.3).

By 1960 the federal share had declined by 6 percentage points to an all-time low of 16 percent, while the private share rose by the same amount to an all-time high of 84 percent. Since industry's share had declined slightly, the nonprofit sector had absorbed the whole of this gain. Higher education increased its share somewhat, but the non-university research centers increased their role as performers as well.

By 1965 other performing sectors made measurable contributions. Government performed 18 percent of the research, but the increase over 1960 was due to the 2 percentage points now recorded for state and local government. The for-profit sector (industry) declined by 7 percentage points from 1960, while the share of the nonprofit sector reached its highest relative level (53 percent). Foreign performers were responsible for 3 percent.

Higher education has long been the principal performer of biomedical research, although it depends almost exclusively on external funding for its research programs. In the pre–World War II years, basic medical research was centered in a few research universities, which also performed most of the modest clinical research. During the war the key agencies of the federal government, particularly the departments of War and Navy, and the Office of Scientific Research and Development (under Bush) had learned to work well with most of the universities with which they had participated on national defense projects. After the war it seemed mutually desirable that these relationships be continued. Although most of the researchers expected to return to the more conventional pattern of academic life, in which they would both teach and perform research, they welcomed the federal grants, which assured center place for the universities.

There were advantages to the federal government in making most of its external grants to universities. As nonprofit enterprises, these required less government surveillance over their use of public dollars. Further, universities were in a position to cooperate in preparing grant requests and in accounting for the money spent and work performed. Finally, by relying on universities to perform much of the total biomedical research, the federal government could expand its funding without having to provide facilities and equipment *de novo* since the university infrastructure was already in place (fig. 2.3).

With the passage of time public support for biomedical research was strengthened by the growing efforts of the Association of American Medical Colleges to assure that the flow of research funds to medical schools be maintained and, whenever possible,

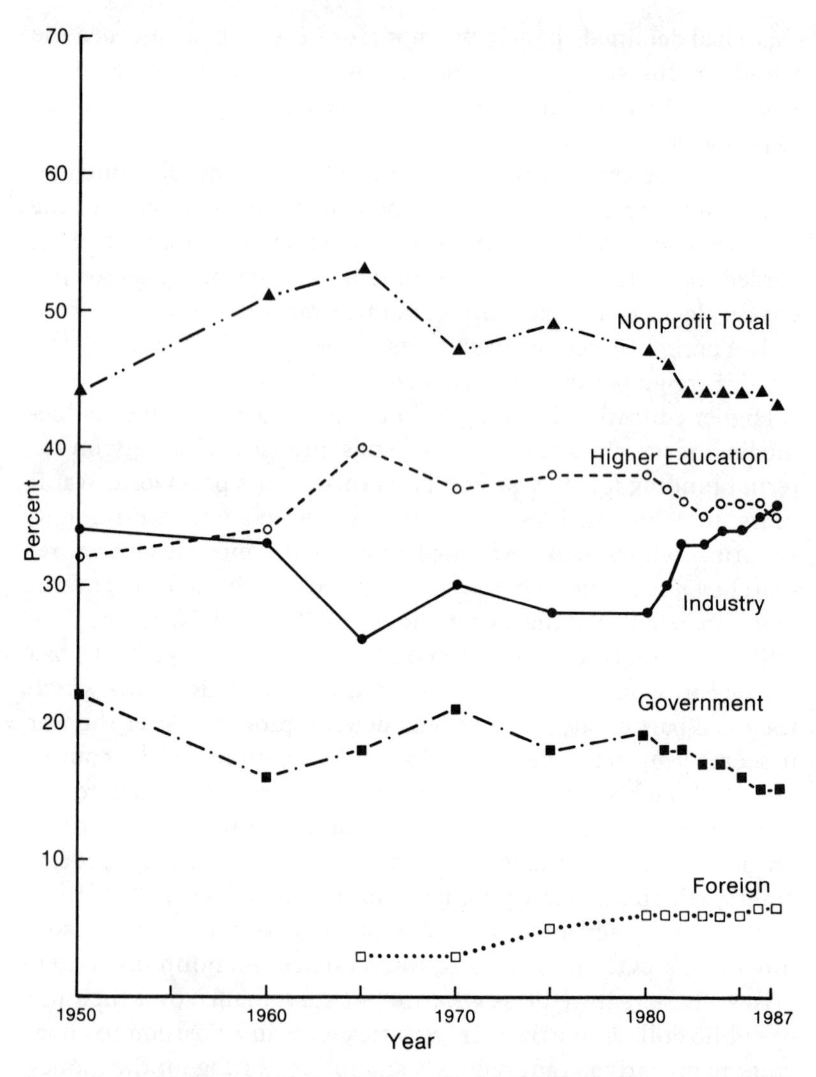

Figure 2.3 Performers of National Biomedical R & D as Percentages of Total, 1950–1987
Source: Table 2.3.

enlarged. In 1969, despite the fact that Chicago had long been the home of the major organizational components of the medical establishment, the association relocated its headquarters to Washington, D.C. to be closer to the scene of action.

As the flow of federal funds to medical schools increased until they accounted for over one-half of the total revenues of the major research centers in the late 1960s, the presidents of these prestigious institutions added their voices to those of others who emphasized the important national goals that could be achieved through continuing strong congressional support for biomedical research.

The established major research-oriented universities, primarily on the east coast, as well as a few newer schools mostly on the west coast, set about expanding staff and facilities to be better positioned to compete for the ever-growing pool of federal dollars. This expansion was for the most part financed by federal grants. The universities thus embarked upon a continuing process of expanding and improving their infrastructures, largely with the dollars that they received from Washington. Since 1948 when the NIH was first authorized to make extramural grants for construction of research facilities, it has expended about $1 billion for the purpose.

The scope of the federal government's role can be better appreciated when one realizes that it made huge sums available for construction and equipment and training grants to increase the supply of future investigators, as well as clinical center grants to enable selected medical schools to explore specialty areas or to strengthen their general clinical research base. For the first fifteen years of enlarged appropriations, 1950–65, the universities and medical schools were often in a catch-up game; the federal government had more money to distribute than the medical centers were capable of absorbing effectively.[6]

Period 2. 1966–1982: Slow Growth

Even if the economic environment had remained favorable, it is unlikely that the high growth rates of the first period would have been maintained. Had this happened, 1987 outlays in constant dollars would have been nine times larger than they actually were. By the early 1960s both the Bureau of the Budget and the Congress had in fact begun to question the effectiveness of continuing to escalate levels of support for biomedical research.

President Johnson also noted that the federal government had supplied about two out of every three dollars for research in the past decade and a half in the hope of achieving significant breakthroughs in medical knowledge and techniques, and that it was time to bring such discoveries as had been made to Americans wherever they lived, even those distant from the centers of medical excellence.

Alternatively, the president noted, if significant breakthroughs from research were not yet imminent, it might be more advisable to redirect federal funds to expanding and improving programs that could improve access to health care for the uninsured and underinsured. In 1967, Congress, at the bidding of the administration, passed the Regional Medical Program, with the aim of speeding the diffusion of recent medical advances from the major educational and research centers to the rest of the country. The program, because of faculty conception, underfunding, and physicians' discontent, moved only haltingly from planning to implementation. Regionalization remained more a goal than a reality because sophisticated medicine required the critical mass of patients and physicians found only in the larger urban centers.

The president was among the earliest to offer cautionary comments about the future level of financing for biomedical research. A few years later, Shannon, after his retirement as director of the NIH, testified before a subcommittee of the U.S. Senate that he was concerned about the future financing of biomedical research because of the growing preoccupation and concern of the Congress with the financing of its two new big and increasingly expensive medical programs, Medicare and Medicaid. Shannon pointed out that, given the dynamics of the political process, particularly the interactions between constituents, who stood to benefit from improved medical care, and members of Congress, who seek to respond to constituents' needs, Congress might be inclined to neglect investments for education and research, the cutting edge that largely determines the long-term status of the nation's health.

It might appear at first that the cautionary comments of President Johnson and Dr. Shannon were unnecessarily pessimistic since total spending for biomedical research in this whole period increased from $1.9 to $9.5 billion in current dollars, a fivefold increase. This was, however, a period characterized by persistent and growing inflation, including four double-digit inflation years (1974, 1979, 1980, and 1981). When current dollars are translated into constant dollars, total outlays increased from $2.7 billion to $4.4 billion, a compounded rate of increase in total funds of only a little more than 3 percent (in contrast to the 16 percent of period

1). In the case of federal funds, the rate of increase had dropped from 18 percent to a little over 2 percent. The funders, particularly the federal government, had stepped hard on the brakes (table 2.4 and fig. 2.4).

By the late 1960s and early 1970s, with the expanded research infrastructure largely in place, federal appropriations in constant dollars had begun to level off. The financial position of the AHCs was shored up in part by the new dollars that began to flow from the large service programs, Medicare and Medicaid, which compensated to some degree for the decrease in funding from the NIH and other federal agencies. Between 1963 and 1976 the flow of federal funds for the expansion of medical school facilities and for increased student enrollments provided yet additional sources of support for medical schools.

During the years of steadily increasing appropriations, the NIH encountered few problems both in providing continuing support to investigators whom it had funded earlier and also in funding new young researchers. But as research dollars became scarcer, it became increasingly difficult for the NIH to fund both groups. The growing stringency in funding is indicated by the ability of the NIH to fund almost three-fifths of all approved competing

Table 2.4 Percentage Annual Change in National Funds for Biomedical R & D, 1950–1987

	Current	Constant
1950	14	7
1955	11	9
1960	25	25
1965	17	15
1970	8	3
1975	11	4
1980	11	3
1981	9	−2
1982	9	2
1983	12	6
1984	13	9
1985	12	8
1986	9	5
1987	11	6

Source: Table 2.1.

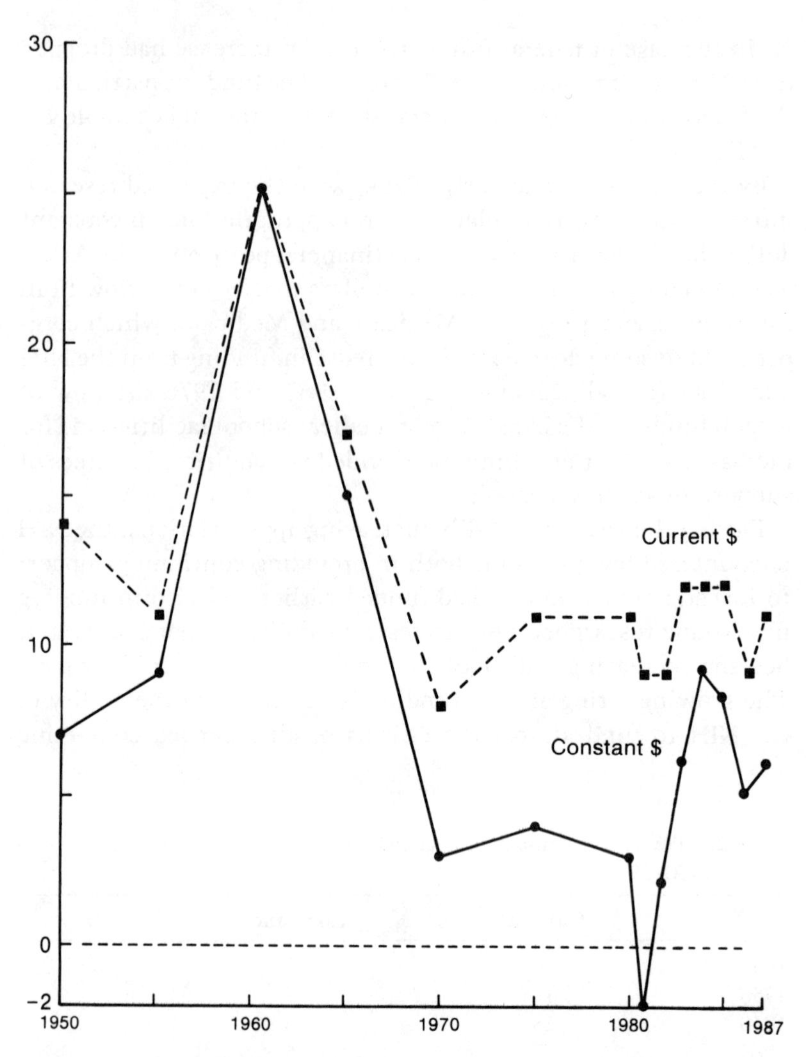

Figure 2.4 Percentage Change in National Funds for Biomedical R & D, 1950–1987
Source: Table 2.4.

projects in the early 1970s but only slightly above one-third a decade later (table 2.5 and fig. 2.5).

The more constrained financial environment for federal funding of research in this period led to other strains. At the beginning of the 1970s, President Nixon declared a "war on cancer" to be fought through increased funds to the National Cancer Institute.

Table 2.5 Percentage of Eligible NIH Competing Research Projects Funded, 1970–1986

	Award Rate		Award Rate
1970	50	1979	52
1971	51	1980	42
1972	59	1981	39
1973	39	1982	35
1974	58	1983	37
1975	61	1984	37
1976	48	1985	37
1977	39	1986	36
1978	45		

Source: U.S. Department of Health and Human Services, National Institutes of Health, *NIH Data Book* (Bethesda, Md., annual).

In 1971 the allocation for the institute amounted to $170 million. The following year it had risen to almost $400 million, and in 1976 the institute received over one-third of all NIH appropriations. The status of the institute within the NIH also changed; its director became a presidential appointee, and its budget had to be transmitted to the president's Office of Management and Budget without change by the NIH or the Department of Health, Education, and Welfare.[7]

Some of the increased funding for cancer research came at the expense of the other institutes, which, as might have been expected, took objection to the reallocation. They argued strongly that nobody could foretell where the breakthroughs in cancer would originate and that a broad-based biomedical research program held greater promise than a narrow concentration on cancer research alone. The critics won their point because in the following years the National Cancer Institute's share of the total NIH grants dropped steadily until by 1987 it stood at 23 percent and the institute was one of the few whose appropriations in current dollars had declined between 1980 and 1982. In constant dollars appropriations for it have still not recovered to the 1977 level (table 2.6 and fig. 2.6).

There were other untoward developments. In 1976 and 1977 the NIH was still able to make about $23 million a year available for the construction of research facilities at universities and medical schools. In the first four years of the 1980s, however, construction

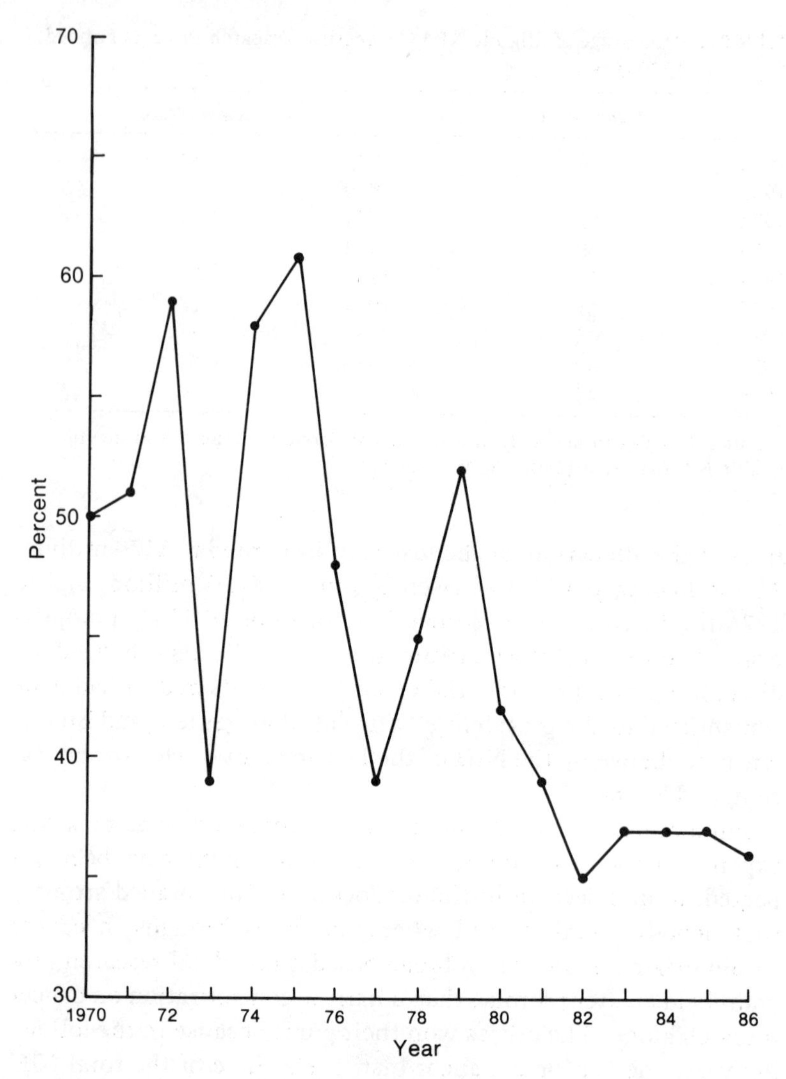

Figure 2.5 Percentages of Eligible NIH Competing Research Projects Funded, 1970–1986
Source: Table 2.5.

allocations amounted to only $5 million, a decline of more than 75 percent.

Another indicator of the impact of more constrained federal funding on research was the stability in the average size of NIH research awards during the late 1970s and early 1980s. Despite

Table 2.6 Percentages of Total NIH Obligations Allocated to Major NIH Institutes, 1971–1986

	NCI	NHLBI	NIADDK	NIGMS
1971	19	16	11	13
1972	25	16	10	11
1973	28	17	9	10
1974	29	16	9	10
1975	33	16	8	9
1976	34	16	8	8
1977	32	15	8	8
1978	31	16	9	8
1979	29	16	10	9
1980	29	15	10	9
1981	28	15	10	9
1982	27	15	10	9
1983	25	16	10	9
1984	24	16	10	9
1985	23	16	11	9
1986	23	17	10	9

Source: U.S. Department of Health and Human Services, National Institutes of Health, *NIH Data Book* (Bethesda, Md., annual).

Note: NCI—National Cancer Institute
NHLBI—National Heart, Lung, and Blood Institute
NIADDK—National Institute of Arthritis, Diabetes, and Digestive and Kidney Diseases
NIGMS—National Institute of General Medical Sciences

the rise in the costs of equipment, materials, and salaries, the size of the traditional award (R01) in constant dollars actually declined between 1977 and 1983 (from $67,400 to $66,600). With the subsequent upswing in federal financing, by 1986 the size of the average award increased to $70,600 in constant dollars.[8]

The relative stability in the size of awards did not reflect the steady rise in the universities' indirect costs from one in five to almost one in three of total grant dollars during the period 1970–1986. Typically, four out of five dollars were formerly used directly by the biomedical investigator; today overhead costs have risen to such an extent that the investigator has access to little more than two out of every three dollars.

Period 3. 1983–1987: Renewed Growth

In 1983 the inflationary spiral was finally brought under control. In that year total current dollar outlays came to $10.5 billion

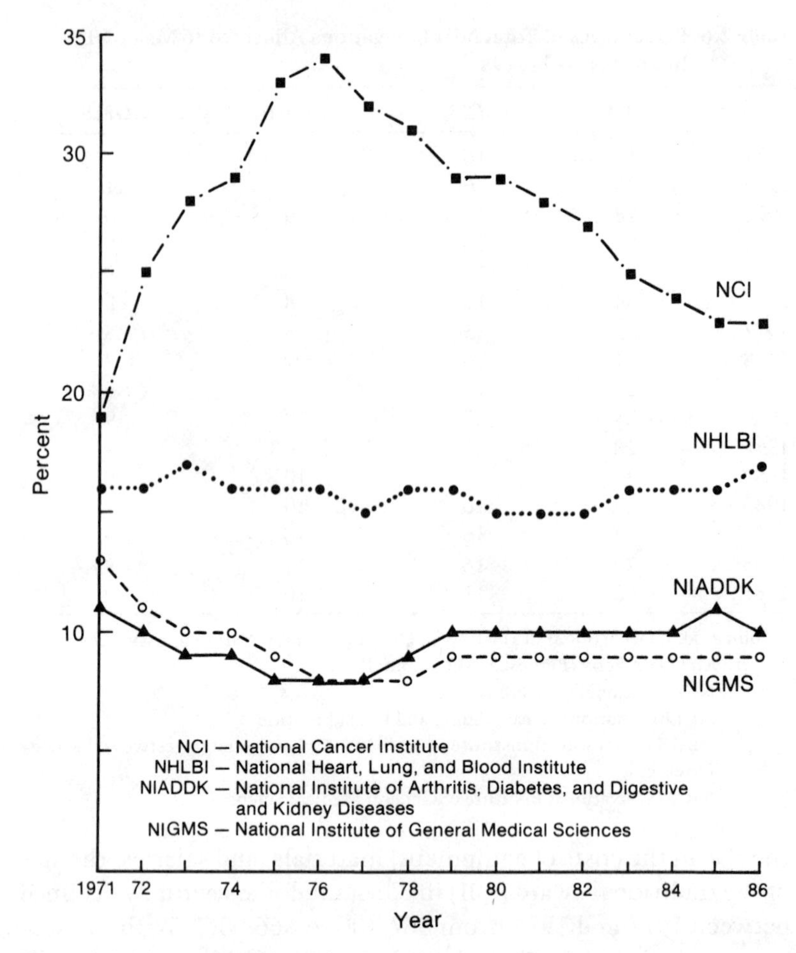

Figure 2.6 Percentages of Total NIH Obligations Allocated to Major NIH Institutes, 1971–1986
Source: Table 2.6.

and the federal share to $5.4 billion, slightly over one-half of the total. In constant dollars total outlays grew from $4.7 to over $6 billion, making for a 7.2 percent rate of increase, almost half the rate of growth of period 1. The rate of increase in federal dollars of only 5 percent explains the declining share of the federal government in this period (from 51 to 47 percent) and the corresponding increase in the share of industry (from 42 to 46 percent).

As the NIH became increasingly aware of the difficulties it confronted in meeting the needs of the biomedical research community in the 1970s as a result of the small increments in its appropriations, it reconsidered its strategy and made two major adjustments, each of which, it believed, would contribute to the more effective use of scarce federal research dollars.

The first adjustment involved the NIH's directing a considerably larger share of its total budget to basic research. In 1970 it directed 44 percent of its budget to the support of basic research whereas in 1987 the proportion had risen to over 60 percent. To accomplish this, the NIH reduced its support for applied research from 39 to 30 percent and for development from about 11 percent to 9 percent (table 2.7 and fig. 2.7).

The other important budgeting shift involved an increase in the proportion of support for research grants from approximately 56 percent in 1977 to 70 percent of its total budget in 1986, even though this required a reduction in its funding for its intramural programs. This was further evidence of the determination of the NIH to fund as many talented investigators as possible within its more restricted budget. The number of research grants was in fact increased by over 50 percent, from about 15,300 to 23,622 in that period.

The recent financial environment has also exacerbated the difficulty of making a speedy response to new situations such as the current epidemic of acquired immune deficiency syndrome (AIDS). In 1982 the Public Health Service obligated about $5.6 million for AIDS, $3.4 million from NIH funds. In 1986 total obligations of the Public Health Service had risen to $234 million, the NIH contribution being $135 million. While some of these enlarged obligations reflected new congressional appropriations,

Table 2.7 Percentage of NIH Funds Allocated to Basic and Applied Research and to Development, 1970–1987

	Basic Research	Applied Research	Development
1970	50.9	38.5	10.6
1975	44.1	41.3	14.7
1980	51.6	36.0	12.4
1986	62.3	29.4	8.3
1987	61.1	29.7	9.2

Sources: National Science Foundation, *Federal Funds for Research and Development: Federal obligations for Research by Agency and Detailed Field of Science, 1967–1986* (Washington, D.C., n.d.); 1987 data from NIH.

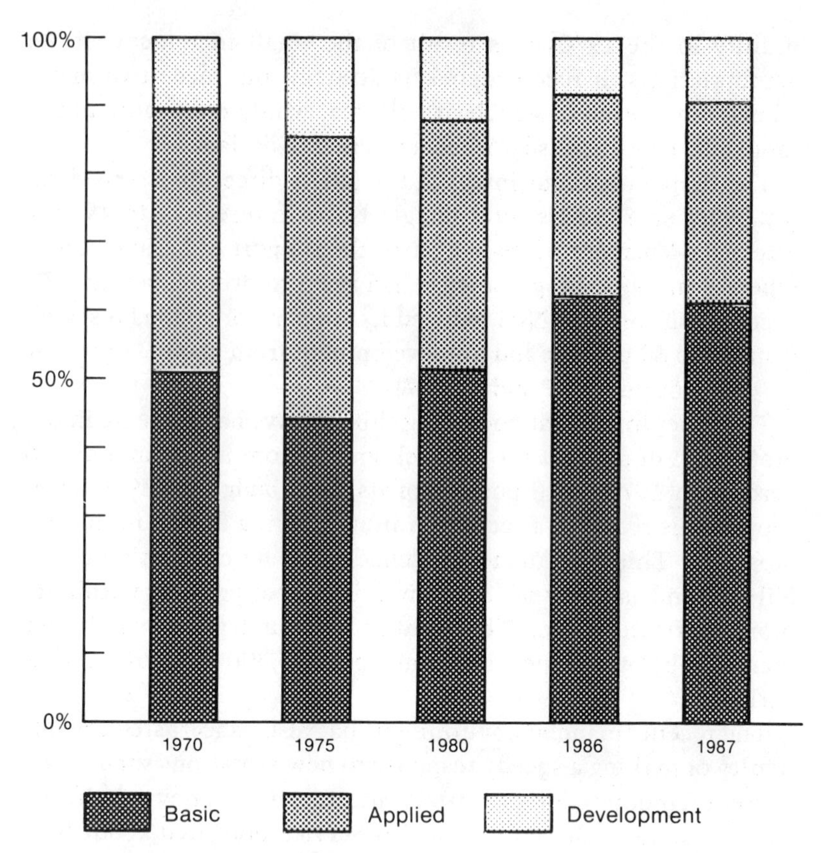

Figure 2.7 Percentage of NIH Funds Allocated to Basic and Applied Research and to Development, 1970–1987
Source: Table 2.7.

a portion involved reallocations from the budgets of the various institutes. The president's budget request for fiscal year 1989 contains a figure of $1.3 billion for AIDS, and increase of 40 percent over 1988.

At the beginning of this decade, several of the important biomedical research institutions explored the possibility of diminishing their dependence on federal funds. Massachusetts General Hospital, Harvard University, Washington University (St. Louis), and Georgetown University were the recipients of large grants or contracts from corporate enterprises that were positioning themselves to move into the expanding arena of biotechnology. For a brief period it appeared as if these efforts were the forerunners of new and continuing sources of funding for universities, AHCs, and other leading nonprofit research institutions. From the vantage of 1988 (the passage of more time may again alter the perspective) it appears that this corporate infusion of research dollars was a one-time effort. There has been little evidence that the experience of the early eighties signified a permanent new large source of funding for basic biomedical research.[9]

The foregoing data about sources and performers of biomedical research and development establishes some of the dimensions of its current structure in the United States and underscores the critical role that the private nonprofit sector, particularly higher education, plays in its performance. Technically speaking, the classification of all higher education in the private nonprofit category, which is NIH practice, is questionable since many of the leading research universities that perform a large part of all biomedical research are state universities and therefore public. However, in recent years most of these institutions, like their private counterparts, have aggressively solicited gifts from alumni, other donors, and organized philanthropy so that the line between them and private nonprofit institutions has become blurred. Similarly, we must consider the appropriateness of the term *private* nonprofit universities, for the largest among them receive annually multimillions of dollars in federal research grants, as well as other forms of governmental aid.

In addition to the difficulties of classifying universities, the data about both the source of funds for and the performance of biomedical research obscure important distinctions between basic research, which is directed to adding to the pool of knowledge, and applied research and development, whose principal aim is the improvement of biomedical products and services. Though there are no fixed criteria to distinguish among the three dimensions of research—basic research, applied research, and development, there is broad agreement that the federal government, mostly through the NIH, is the principal source of funds for, and higher educational institutions are the principal performers of, basic research. Together, universities, medical schools, and a few freestanding private nonprofit institutions are the principal performing sectors of most basic research.

Applied research and development are the principal concerns of industry, which both finances and performs applied biomedical research. In its continuing search to develop improved and new biomedical products and services, industry is limited by the breadth and depth of the extant pool of knowledge, although it should be noted that the unsolved problems researchers face in the applied area often stimulate basic researchers to undertake new lines of inquiry.

Finally, special attention should be directed to clinical research because much of the basic research on biological systems has as its goal the discovery of a cure for or the alleviation of many of the costly and destructive diseases that afflict humans. Unless the knowledge gained from animals in the laboratory can be tested and refined and proves helpful to the patient, it will be stillborn, at least until it serves as a building block for further basic research or another way is found to make it a part of the medical armamentarium.[10]

With the longer perspective of almost four decades, we can present the highlights of the changing patterns in the funding and performance of biomedical research.

—The decision of the federal government in the immediate postwar period to assume the major role in financing basic research catapulted the United States into a position of global leadership in providing sophisticated health care for a part, if not the whole, of its population. Although the liberally financed research programs did not find definitive cures for many of the worst diseases, they contributed greatly to the accumulation of new knowledge and new techniques that were beneficial to the health and well-being of the American people.

—The research-oriented universities, medical schools, institutes, and teaching hospitals (the private nonprofit complex) responded enthusiastically to the new opportunities that the federal funding created. The evolving structure of biomedical research represented in the first instance a loose but effective liaison between the federal government and the institutions of higher education that received most of the external funding of the NIH and other federal agencies.

Quite early in its expansion, as we have shown, the NIH, in association with the academic leadership, decided upon the process of peer review of individual investigators' grant requests as a sound basis for distributing the funds that Congress had appropriated for biomedical research. The key terms are *peer review* and *individual grant* requests.

One could have imagined a government-university relationship in which the former made annual allocations for research to recipient institutions to be subdivided by them among their schools, departments, and faculty members. But such a system would have required that Congress develop an acceptable basis for making such allocations based on the research potential of the competing institutions—no easy matter. The peer review process offered an attractive alternative. It should be noted, however, that the NIH also had authority to make institutional grants over the succeeding decades for construction, training, various types of centers, program support, and still other institutional purposes.

With regard to the impact of increased federal funding for biomedical research in universities, the following are worthy of note: Substantial federal funding led to the development of the AHCs as the preeminent institutions in the health care system and propelled U.S. medical care into a leadership role among the advanced nations; it contributed heavily to tilting the medical educational system toward specialization; it altered the power structure in medical schools away from the deans, who had oversight over the university's allocations, to the chairs of the basic science and clinical departments, who came to control most of the federal money; it shifted the interest and concern of medical schools from the undergraduate training of practitioners to the postgraduate training of specialists; and by encouraging the vast increase in the number of faculty (primarily for research), it made the research-oriented medical schools vulnerable to any leveling off or decline in federal funding. But before these and other significant institutional realignments surfaced, the new structure of biomedical research had become firmly entrenched.

—Industry paralleled the federal government's vastly expanded outlays for research, but its dollars were expended primarily on applied research and development in the hope and expectation of bringing profitable new products and services to the market. It should be observed that industry had ready access to the ever-broader and deeper pool of biomedical knowledge and technology as a result of the federal government's liberal support of basic research.

—Although philanthropic dollars had played a significant role in supporting the modest pre–World War II research efforts, philanthropy's relative position declined soon after the federal government opened its sluice gates. However, philanthropy continued to play a role in the infrastructure of biomedical research through capital grants and endowments.

In the era of accelerated federal funding, between 1950 and 1965, the steady stream of federal dollars dominated the academic scene so that philanthropy no longer saw a significant role for itself in the financing of biomedical research. However, during the last two decades, the hard-pressed academic institutions, which are finding additional governmental dollars harder to attract, have started to reopen their lines to the philanthropic community in the hope that philanthropy can introduce an element of stability in their research environment.

The decision of the federal government in the immediate post–World War II era to become the leading funder of basic and applied research and development left its mark on many of the nation's mainline institutions including industry, the universities, and the research community. Nowhere was its impact greater than in the medical realm, for the external funding by the NIH went far to alter the orientation of the nation's leading medical schools in the direction of laboratory research, vastly increased the number of investigators, and by contributing greatly to the specialization that came to characterize the medical profession, resulted in the dominance of high-tech medicine.

The availability of large new sources of research dollars did not result, as the proponents had hoped, in the discovery of early cures for the most devastating diseases. But it did set the stage for major breakthroughs in molecular biology that hold the greatest promise of leading to those elusive cures.

3 · Investment in Biomedical Research: Critical Ratios

There is nothing simple or straightforward about the absolute or relative amounts of money that national governments or corporations are able and willing to invest in research relative to other areas in which they can employ their available resources. The problem is that much more complicated for governments of advanced nations, which face the competing demands of infrastructure, defense, education, and research and, within the research area itself, among the natural, biological, and social sciences.

Since all investment activity is speculative because the future cannot be foretold, decision makers in the for-profit, nonprofit, and governmental sectors must in the end rely on their best judgment in making investment decisions.

Confronted with this basic dilemma, decision makers have tended to develop various approaches to the collection and analysis of data as a guide to investment decisions.

As we have noted, the federal government moved aggressively after World War II to increase its annual funding for biomedical research in response to a combination of factors that began with the emphasis that President Roosevelt had placed in his letter of 17 November 1944 to Dr. Vannevar Bush.

With particular reference to the war of science against disease, what can be done now to organize a program for continuing in the future the work which has been done in medicine and related sciences?

The fact that the annual deaths in this country from one or two diseases alone are far in excess of the total number of lives lost by us in battle during this war should make us conscious of the duty we owe future generations.[1]

The Bush report made the following critical points:

—Progress in the war against disease depends upon a flow of new scientific knowledge.
—The responsibility for basic research . . . falls primarily upon the medical schools and the universities.
—The traditional sources of support for medical research . . . are diminishing
—If we are to maintain the progress in medicine which has marked the last 25 years, the Government should extend financial support to basic medical research.
—The amount which can be effectively spent in the first year should not exceed 5 million dollars. After a program is under way perhaps 20 million dollars a year can be spent effectively.[2]

A close reading of the report indicates that the absence of large philanthropic gifts during the depressed decade of the 1930s led to the perception that the future of medical school finances was a precarious one. Only government support could assure the level of basic research in biology and medicine essential to the discovery of cures for the major killer diseases. It was clear to President Roosevelt, to Dr. Bush, and to the distinguished members of his advisory committee that the federal government must support basic research or forgo the advances that could lead to lower morbidity, and an improvement in the quality of life of the citizenry.

The $20 million of annual support that Bush recommended for the program after it had become established must be considered against the background of a total federal outlay for biomedical research (largely for intramural use) of $3 million in 1940. It is well known that most new federal programs command only small initial appropriations. By 1947, however, the total federal outlay for biomedical research already stood at $27 million, and by 1950 it had risen to $74 million.

The huge expansion thereafter, as well as its ebbs and flows, reflected the pull of different opinions on the "right" amount to spend for biomedical research. In the give-and-take of the government's and industry's budgetary processes, liberal and conservative proponents alike fall back on the use of "critical ratios" to buttress their positions. No one critical ratio commands general acceptance, and legislators and business people alike are prone at different times to use those that support their current preferences.

The better-known ratios advanced since Bush's modest budgetary proposal will be reviewed briefly.

The Ratio of Total Expenditures for Biomedical Research and Development to Total Population

One widely used ratio measures total expenditures for biomedical research relative to the total population or research dollars per capita. In 1950 this ratio in current dollars came to $1.02 per person per year. In 1987 the comparable figure was $66.58, a sixty-fivefold increase. In constant dollars, the gain was a still striking twelvefold increase.[3]

While an increase of this magnitude speaks to a major national effort to broaden the support of biomedical research, it must be placed in the context of the rapid economic growth of the quarter-century following the end of World War II. Such an economic environment permitted both national investment and consumer spending to rise simultaneously. Moreover, the steeply rising ratio reflected a response to the new opportunities created by the enlarged pool of knowledge and the significant technological breakthroughs to which it led.

Table 3.1 reveals that since 1970 there has been stability, not increase, in the nation's outlay for biomedical research when both biomedical research and GNP expressed in constant dollars are measured on a per capita basis. The large gains had occurred in the earlier period of rapid growth, between 1950 and 1970.

Given the small investment per capita in biomedical research relative to the size of the nation's GNP one might conclude that a larger outlay for biomedical research is justified. But the GNP is not a resource pool that is under the exclusive control of the federal government. Households control the largest segment, business another significant segment.

Of a total GNP of $4.5 trillion in 1987, the federal government's budget is about $1 trillion. But this does not mean that the federal government has broad discretion about how to spend this huge sum. Most of its revenue is committed to interest payments, entitlement programs, and urgent defense requirements. Looked

Table 3.1 Ratio of per Capita Expenditures for Biomedical R & D to per Capita GNP
(In Constant $)

	GNP per Capita	Biomedical R & D per Capita	Ratio (%)
1950	3,406	2.09	0.06
1970	5,073	14.56	0.29
1980	6,498	18.38	0.28
1986	7,595	23.76	0.31
1987	7,889	25.33	0.32

Source: Eli Ginzberg and Anna B. Dutka, *The Financing of Biomedical Research in the United States, 1950–1985. A Chartbook and Text* (Conservation of Human Resources, Columbia University, March 1986), mimeograph; 1986 and 1987 data added.

at from the perspective of discretionary expenditures, that is, items in the budget over which the Congress has some degree of freedom of action, the figure for federal spending of $7.6 billion for biomedical research is not insignificant.

The Ratio of Total Federal Expenditures for Biomedical Research and Development to Total Federal Outlays

Because of the significant role that the federal government has played in the financing of biomedical research throughout the entire postwar era, it is desirable to look at another critical ratio—that between total federal expenditures for biomedical research and the total outlays of the federal government. Table 3.2 sets out the key ratios for selected years.

Between 1950 and 1965, when total federal outlays expanded somewhat less than threefold, federal outlays for biomedical research increased sixteen fold, bringing the ratio of federal expenditures for biomedical research to total federal outlays in 1965 to the 1 percent level for the first time. From then on, the ratio declined, reflecting the more rapid growth of total federal outlays for other functions.

Two additional ratios focus on more specific areas of federal involvement in the biomedical research area.

Table 3.2 Ratio of Total Federal Expenditures for Biomedical R & D to Total Federal Outlays
(In Current $ Billions)

	Total Federal Outlays	Total Federal Expenditures for Biomedical R & D	Ratio (%)
1950	42	0.07	0.2
1965	118	1.2	1.0
1980	591	4.5	0.8
1986	980	7.2	0.7
1987 (estimated)	1,015	7.6	0.7

Source: Eli Ginzberg and Anna B. Dutka, *The Financing of Biomedical Research in the United States, 1950–1985. A Chartbook and Text* (Conservation of Human Resources, Columbia University, March 1986), mimeograph; 1986 and 1987 data added.

The Ratio of Federal Expenditures for Biomedical Research and Development to the Total Federal Budget for Research and Development

In 1950 biomedical research represented 5.6 percent of the total. By the end of the 1960s it had almost doubled, and by 1980 it reached a high point of 15.6 percent, almost a threefold gain over 1950. Clearly, Congress had decided to favor biomedical research over many competing claims for federal dollars.

In the 1980s the federal government increased its total R & D budget from $30 billion to over $58 billion primarily by increasing the budgetary authority of the Department of Defense by about $28 billion.[4] Biomedical research also experienced a substantial increase, from $4.7 billion in 1980 to $7.6 billion in 1987. The proportion that biomedical research expenditures represented of total federal R & D expenditures in 1987 stood at 13 percent.[5] This means that of every eight dollars that the federal government invests in R & D across the entire scientific gamut, one dollar is made available to push back the biological and medical frontiers.

The Ratio of Federal Basic Research Expenditures to Total National Basic Research Expenditures

If our concern is concentrated solely on investment in basic research in all disciplines, we find that in 1987 total national support for basic research amounted to $14.8 billion, of which the federal government accounted for $8.8 billion, 60 percent of the total. Government's large share is not surprising since basic research is a risky investment undertaken for the long-term public good, not the type of investment that the for-profit sector usually undertakes with stockholders' money.[6]

Although the 1970s and the 1980s were difficult years marked by accelerating inflation and three recessions, two of them serious, basic research fared relatively well. Between 1970 and 1985 total expenditures for basic research increased from $3.6 billion to $13.3 billion, almost fourfold in current dollars and by 46 percent in constant dollars.

In 1987, with total federal obligations for basic research amounting to over $8.8 billion in current dollars, the NIH with almost $3.4 billion accounted for 39 percent, the largest share. The National Science Foundation, the departments of Defense and Energy, and the National Aeronautics and Space Administration followed in that order.

The Ratios of National and Federal Expenditures for Biomedical Research and Development to National and Federal Total Expenditures for Health Care

Possibly the most significant critical ratios relate national and federal expenditures for biomedical research to national and federal expenditures for health care. These ratios in effect relate the investment share of total health spending, as measured by expenditures for biomedical research, to the current operating expenditures for health care services.

In 1965, the year before Medicare and Medicaid became operational, the total health care expenditures of the United States (including $1.9 billion for the construction of health-related facilities and almost $1.9 billion for biomedical research) amounted to $41.9 billion. The sums expended on biomedical research accounted for 4.5 percent of these outlays.

Table 3.3 Ratios of National and Federal Expenditures for Biomedical R & D to National and Federal Total Expenditures for Health, 1965–1987
(In Current $ Millions)

	National Expenditures			Federal Expenditures		
	Biomedical R & D	Total Health	Ratio (%)	Biomedical R & D	Total Health	Ratio (%)
1965	1,884	41,900	4.5	1,174	5,625	21.0
1975	4,701	132,673	3.3	2,832	37,079	7.6
1985	13,346	422,600	3.2	4,723	65,762	7.2
1986	14,605	458,200	3.2	6,895	126,622	5.5
1987 estimated	16,180	496,600	3.3	7,640	142,700	5.4

Sources: U.S. Department of Health and Human Services, Health Care Financing Administration, *Health Care Financing Review* (Washington, D.C., annual); and National Institutes of Health, *NIH Data Book* (Bethesda, Md., annual).

As table 3.3 reveals, although funding for biomedical research continued to increase, total outlays for health care increased more rapidly.

The decline in the ratio of expenditures for biomedical research to total health care outlays after Medicare and Medicaid were implemented confirms the opinion voiced earlier by James Shannon that, in the competition for dollars between research and service entitlement programs, research was likely to lose ground.

If the focus is shifted to federal outlays for health care, the impact of the new entitlement programs is even more striking. In 1965 the federal government's expenditures for all health activities was about $5.6 billion, which included health care benefits for its civilian employees, health services provided to the military and their dependents, the health and hospital activities of the Veterans Administration, and the outlays of the Public Health Service, which included most of the $1.2 billion that the federal government made available for biomedical research and development. Research absorbed about 21 percent of all federal expenditures for health care. By 1975 the research share had declined to less than 8 percent, and in 1985 to about 7 percent. The Congressional Budget Office's analysis of the president's budget for 1988 shows a total of $119 billion for the two major health care programs: Function 550 (health—Medicaid, Public Health Service, and Federal Employees' Health Benefits), which amounts to $41 billion, and Function 570 (Medicare), which will cost $78 billion.[7] To this must be added over $10 billion for the health services provided veterans and $9 billion for those for members of the armed forces and their dependents. In short, the total expenditures of the federal government for health care in fiscal year 1988 can be expected to exceed those of previous years. Since it is problematic whether the total federal outlay for biomedical research will exceed $8 billion, it is likely that the ratio of research funds to total federal outlays for health will decline further.

In its analysis of the president's budget proposal, the Congressional Budget Office noted: "The Administration proposes to cap spending for the Public Health Service at the 1987 level. This action would result in savings over five years of $10.7 billion below the CBO baseline. Most of this reduction is achieved through limiting research funding for the National Institutes of Health."[8]

The introductory statement to this section warrants emphasis. "The President requests sharp cuts in the health area, capping both federal Medicaid and Public Health Service spending. Most of the proposals have been submitted by the President in previous budgets and have not been approved by the Congress."[9]

It is clear that in 1965, when more than one out of every five federal dollars spent for health was allocated to research, the support of biomedical research was a key facet of the federal government's expenditures for health. But in recent years, because of the heavy financial burden imposed by the rising costs of Medicare and the partial financing of Medicaid, the federal government has reduced sharply its relative share (though not the absolute amount) of its funding for research. Currently one out of every sixteen federal dollars spent on health is allocated to biomedical research.

The obvious competition between federal support for service programs and federal support for biomedical research is revealed by the figures: if the government had maintained the 1965 ratio between research and total health outlays, the 1988 appropriation for federal research would be $29 billion, rather than the $8 billion that appears probable.

The search for critical ratios requires that attention also be given to industry, which currently accounts for about 42 percent of all outlays for biomedical research, making this source second in size only to the federal government.

The Ratio of Industry's Research and Development to Sales

The point has been made that federal investments in biomedical research, and in particular for basic research, provide a favorable environment for industry to enlarge its own outlays so that new or improved products and services may be marketed. Clearly, the growth and vitality of the U.S. pharmaceutical industry depend in no small measure on the ability and willingness of the federal government to pursue a broad-based policy for supporting biomedical research. Without such support and without the parallel contribution of higher education, which trains the many scientists and researchers that industry hires, the pharmaceutical sector would not have been able to achieve its strong competitive position. This is not to say that the relationship between the academic community and industry has been uniform.

Research interactions between academe and industry grew rapidly during the 1920s, 1930s, and early 1940s. By the end of World War II a National Research Council survey revealed that over 300 companies representing a variety of industries were supporting research in universities through fellowships, scholarships, and direct grants-in-aid. Of these firms, nearly 50 were subsidizing over 270 biomedical research projects at about 70 universities. A few universities, such as Cornell, Harvard, Cincinnati, and New York University, led the rest of the group in total projects funded by companies, but by and large the support (which amounted to a minimum of $400,000–500,000) was spread fairly evenly among all the schools.

In the decades following World War II, despite the birth of some novel forms of interaction at a handful of academic institutions, such as Stanford, MIT, and North Carolina, contacts between academe and industry slowly weakened, eventually reaching their nadir by the early 1970s. Some authorities on science and technology policy have blamed this decreasing level of collaborative research at least partially for the decline of American industrial innovation. Several reasons account for this change. First, the post-World War II era witnessed the rise of mega-support for academic research by the federal government. Consequently, university researchers had less incentive to engage in work for industry. In particular, the support that federal defense and aerospace agencies offered to academic scientists led more and more of the latter to focus on the "performance improvements" of high technology rather than the "cost improvements" of other industrial research. Second, as more federal funds filled university research coffers and as higher education in general expanded in the post-war years, graduate students increasingly lost interest in careers in industrial research. Faculty appointments seemed more promising than in the past, and professors began training their students primarily for positions in academe. Finally, industry's involvement in basic research declined. Firms supported less basic research in universities after the mid-1950's, which eroded an important point of contact for academic and industrial scientists.

In the late 1970s and early 1980s, however, links between academe and industry were on the rise again.[10]

The R & D activities of the U.S. pharmaceutical companies account for the major part of all industry outlays for biomedical research. In 1983 the R & D expenditures of U.S. companies that manufacture ethical drugs for human use amounted to $3.1 billion, or 80 percent of the total $3.9 billion industry investment in research. The remaining 20 percent reflected primarily outlays by the chemical, electronics, and professional and scientific instruments industries for biotechnology, imaging and lasers, ultrasound, and the like.

Between 1983 and 1986 total industry outlays for biomedical research increased some 18 percent from $3.9 billion to $4.6 billion. According to the testimony presented to the Subcommittee on Health of the House Committee on Ways and Means by the executive vice president of the Pharmaceutical Manufacturers Association, the pharmaceutical industry alone would invest $5 billion in R & D in 1987.[11]

The ratios between R & D spending on ethical drugs by U.S. pharmaceutical companies and their worldwide sales amounted to 9.2 percent in 1970, 8.9 percent in 1980, and 12.9 percent in 1983. The industry's sales increased fourfold between 1970 and 1983 in current dollars, while its R & D outlays increased 5.5-fold.[12]

There are marked differences in the ratios of the sales of ethical drugs to total sales among the principal U.S. pharmaceutical companies. In the early 1980s, Merck headed the list, with 79 percent of its total sales accounted for by sales of ethical drugs, while

Johnson and Johnson was lowest, with only 25 percent. This difference in the product mixes of these companies is generally correlated with the percentage of sales revenues that they invest in R & D. Those that are more heavily concentrated in the production of pharmaceuticals tend to spend between 8 and 10 percent or even more on R & D, whereas those that focus on consumer products spend considerably less. Across the board, the sixteen largest U.S. pharmaceutical companies spend on average about 7 percent of their sales revenues on R & D.[13]

Research and Development by Industry: Other Aspects

During the last years the U.S. pharmaceutical companies have called attention to a number of trends that they view as ominous for themselves as well as for the future position of the United States in the global market. The United States continues to have the largest ethical drug market, but on a per capita basis Japan has a larger market and the four largest West European nations—West Germany, France, Italy, and the United Kingdom—have a combined market equal to that of the United States.[14] These six countries account for more than one-half of the world's market of ethical drugs. The *Financial Times* of London recently estimated the annual revenues of the pharmaceutical industry worldwide at $100 billion and went on to point out that they have been growing at 5–10 percent a year over the past decade.[15]

The U.S. companies have also called attention to the marked decline in the years of effective life of a patent between the mid-1960s and the early 1980s. In 1965 the figure stood at 15.8 years, in 1975 at 10.4, and in 1982 (the latest year for which data are available) at 9.7, a decline of 39 percent within a period of less than two decades. The industry ascribes this reduction primarily to tighter rules governing the licensing of new products after the patent has been obtained, particularly the size and length of clinical trials that must be completed and reviewed before the Food and Drug Administration will validate a drug as both safe and beneficial for public use.[16]

A recent analysis in *Health Affairs* of developments in the pharmaceutical industry pointed out that "the cost to develop and gain market approval for a new product has risen significantly, along with the time necessary to complete the process . . . A recent study indicates that the cost is $125 million (1986 dollars) to bring a single new product to market. For the drugs approved by the FDA in 1986—the development and approval time on average exceeded ten years . . . Forty-seven new products were introduced worldwide in 1986. The U.S. and Japan are the leading countries in drug innovation with traditional U.S. leadership receiving a strong challenge from Japan."[17]

The more rigid regulatory requirements governing the introduction of new drugs in the United States was one of several reasons why the U.S. pharmaceutical industry has shifted more of its R & D dollars abroad. If it operated through an independent subsidiary, it could escape the tight surveillance of the Food and Drug Administration. Between 1970 and 1983 total R & D investments in constant dollars of U.S. companies marketing ethical pharmaceuticals increased by 115 percent. However, the annual growth rate in the United States amounted to 5.1 percent while the annual rate of investment overseas was 12.8 percent, 2.5 times that in the United States.[18]

Though tighter regulation provides part of the explanation, several other factors are involved. During this period, U.S. companies increased the proportion of their total sales in foreign markets from under one-third to over two-fifths. Multinationals find it desirable to perform both R & D and manufacturing in their major foreign markets to attest to the importance that they attach to their presence in these markets. Further, many U.S. firms have found it desirable to tap into the pool of able foreign scientists. And finally, some countries such as Ireland offer attractive tax benefits.

The foreign share of R & D expenditures funded by U.S. industry rose from 8.4 percent in 1970 to a high of 21.8 percent in 1980. Since that time the proportion has declined to 18.5 percent, still more than twice the 1970 level.

The counterpoint to this development has been a continuing increase in the number of U.S. patents granted to drugs and medicine of foreign origin. Of the 1,114 U.S. drug patents issued in 1970, 62 percent were of U.S. origin, with only 1 percent owned by foreigners. Of the 38 percent of patents of foreign origin, almost one-quarter (10 percent of the total) were granted to U.S. companies with foreign laboratories. In 1981, when the total number of patents granted had increased to 2,596, those of U.S. origin had dropped to 50 percent. There had also been a decrease in U.S. ownership of patents of foreign origin from 10 to 6 percent.

There are other significant aspects of the role of industry in the financing of biomedical research. It must be remembered that for the most part industry spends its R & D funds overwhelmingly for applied research and development and only a small amount for basic research. However, in 1986 industry—primarily the pharmaceutical companies—increased its total R & D spending to $5.7 billion, which began to approximate the $7.2 billion outlay of the federal government for biomedical research in that year. In 1965 the federal government accounted for 62 percent of the nation's biomedical research effort and industry for 24 percent. Since then, as we have shown, a dramatic shift has occurred, until by 1987 the federal share had dropped below 50 percent and industry's share had risen to 42 percent.

This review of trends in critical ratios relating to investment in biomedical research since World War II indicates the following:

—There was a twelvefold increase in constant dollars in per capita spending for biomedical research.

—Large increases in federal spending for R & D were accompanied by a parallel increase in the share going to basic research, which doubled.

—The federal government, the principal source of funds for basic R & D, has made a special effort in recent years to increase further its support for basic research.

—Federal support for biomedical research rose substantially between 1950 and 1965, when it peaked at 1 percent of total federal expenditures. Although this ratio declined subsequently, it remains at approximately 0.75 percent.

—In 1965, the year before Medicare and Medicaid legislation was implemented, biomedical research accounted for 4.5 percent of total national health care outlays. In 1987 it was estimated to stand at 3 percent of the total.

—The establishment and expansion of these two large medical entitlement programs radically reduced the research share of total federal health care outlays from 21 to 6 percent.

—Industry has significantly increased its funding for biomedical research in the last two decades and now accounts for almost

42 percent of the total, only 5 percentage points below the level of the federal government.

—The pharmaceutical companies have recently increased their R & D expenditures, both in absolute terms and as a percentage of their sales.

—A growing proportion of the U.S. pharmaceutical companies' sales are in foreign countries, and these companies have increased their R & D abroad at a faster rate than they have in the United States.

—As a result of tighter federal regulations, there has been a significant decline in the effective length of patent life, which has made it costlier and riskier for industry to invest in R & D. Worldwide competition, however, has left the leading companies no option but to diversify and to increase their investments in research.

—The number of new patents of U.S. origin granted for new drug products has declined over the last two decades to a point where the United States accounts for only slightly more than one-half of all new patents.

Though the critical ratios that have been reviewed shed light on different aspects of the U.S. investment in biomedical research over the last decades, these cannot by themselves reveal whether the nation is pursuing an optimal investment policy. Chapter 4 explores the difficulties of determining how much money an affluent, forward-looking society such as ours "should" spend on biomedical research.

4 · How Many Dollars Are Enough?

Vannevar Bush's report of 1945 contained a recommendation that the federal government aim at an eventual annual expenditure of $20 million for biomedical research. An outlay of between $5 million and $7 million was proposed for the initial years, but the report noted that as the program developed, a larger sum might be required. The point of recalling these early estimates is to underscore that the experts of that day had no way to gauge the effective absorptive capacity of a tremendously expanded research establishment that had not yet been put in place.

There are other reasons why these early estimates proved to be at variance with later developments. The experts looked at only one side of the equation, the expanded role of financing by the federal government. They were concerned primarily with future funding for basic research and only to a lesser degree with total outlays for biomedical research because they believed that funding for basic research fell within the special province of the federal government.

The deficiencies of the many critical ratios we reviewed should serve as a reminder that no single criterion can provide adequate guidance to legislators in determining the appropriate level of investment in research, in the biomedical or any other arena.

Though each ratio may be suggestive, in the last analysis legislators, like business people, must make trade-offs in deciding between spending more on current operations or investing in research. Moreover, Congress must also judge the proportion of its research dollars that should be put into the competing areas of defense, energy, space, the environment, and health, all of which hold promise of contributing to the public welfare.

In 1945, Bush had supported the recommendation for a federal "war against disease" in these terms:

The death rate for all diseases in the Army, including the overseas forces, has been reduced from 14.1 per thousand in the last war to 0.6 per thousand in this war.

Such ravaging diseases as yellow fever, dysentery, typhus, tetanus, pneumonia, and meningitis have been all but conquered by penicillin and the sulfa drugs, the insecticide DDT, better vaccines, and improved hygienic measures. Malaria has been controlled. There has been dramatic progress in surgery.

The striking advances in medicine during the war have been possible only because we had a large backlog of scientific data accumulated through basic research in many scientific fields in the years before the war.[1]

Bush also called attention to many other advances, emphasizing again that *"progress in combating disease depends upon an expanding body of new scientific knowledge."*[2] For the better part of two decades after V-J Day, Congress passed ever-larger appropriations for biomedical research, which indicated its belief that the expansion of the pool of basic knowledge was yielding and would continue to yield significant dividends to the American people by reducing morbidity and mortality. Congress did not ask hard questions about the "rate of return" from this steadily increasing federal investment in research. Its members knew that U.S. scientists were winning Nobel prizes for physiology and medicine; that advances in diagnosis and therapy were adding to the quality of life of many who were stricken by disease or were handicapped or impaired; and that U.S. medicine was preeminent among all nations.

In 1976, Julius H. Comroe, Jr. and Robert D. Dripps published an insightful historical analysis of the effects of earlier research on recent advances in the treatment of cardiovascular diseases which was published in two volumes the following year.[3] They concluded that many of the new treatments depended on long-forgotten basic research across a wide spectrum of the natural sciences. To adopt Robert Merton's felicitous phrase, work was carried out "on the shoulders of giants" (and also on the shoulders of many mundane research workers). Congress accepted the hypothesis that enlarging the pool of basic knowledge would more than pay for itself. However, as Comroe and Dripps found, the time from new knowledge to useful applications could be long, sometimes very long. The following were among the most important findings that Comroe and Dripps extracted from their review of 663 articles critical to the ten top clinical advances in cardiovascular diseases:

—More than two out of five investigators pursued a goal that at the time was unrelated to later clinical advance.
—Over three out of five articles reported on basic research performed to determine mechanisms by which living organisms (including humans) function or by which drugs act.
—Over two-thirds of the research was undertaken in colleges, universities, medical schools, and associated hospitals.
—The lag between initial discovery and effective clinical application was: for about 8 percent, less than 1 year; for 18 percent, 1–10 years; for 17 percent, 11–20 years; for 39 percent, 21–50 years; only (*sic*) 18 percent required more than 50 years.
—Since a high proportion of key research is done by relatively few scientists, the authors recommended "that the NIH regard its *finding* function as important as its *funding* function," giving the highest priority "to the early *finding* of creative individuals and later to long-term, secure funding for their research on their own ideas" (emphasis in original).

In 1970, Robert W. Berliner, then a senior administrator at the NIH, together with his colleague Thomas J. Kennedy, reviewed the various bases used by the Congress to determine "National Expenditures for Biomedical Research." Berliner raised the issue at a time when the earlier free-spending era was clearly coming to an end.[4]

In their thoughtful presentation to the Association of American Medical Colleges, Berliner and Kennedy noted that those persons charged with allocating federal funds were not oblivious to the research and teaching needs of the medical schools and the universities, nor to the critical role that health manpower plays in both the performance of medical research and the provision of medical services to the population. The heart of their presentation, however, explored the theoretical basis for aggregate funding levels.

They called attention to a number of alternative bases. The first holds that R & D is a necessary "overhead on the GNP" and ties the national investment in research to the growth of the GNP. The concept of biomedical research as "overhead on medical care expenditures" was then considered. Berliner and Kennedy observed that "the costs that the health system has been spared as a result of the development of viral vaccines (as for polio, rubella, measles); innovations in antibiotic chemotherapy . . . and the introduction of psychoactive drugs . . . alone exceed by far the total investment since 1940 in biomedical research."[5]

They explored three additional approaches—the effective utilization of available manpower, planned and regular growth, and cost-benefit economics—each of which they found lacking. Setting the level of research so that all available manpower is utilized "carries unacceptable elements of positive feedback; there is no empirical support for the explicitly proposed exponent for growth; and measures of the gains from health research in the form of lives saved and pain reduced or eliminated are elusive. There is no answer possible in the framework of economic investment theory."[6]

Berliner and Kennedy end by favoring "disjointed opportunistic incrementalism," which recognizes that the federal government does not develop a new budget each year from a zero base. Since 1945 a complex system and network for biomedical research has been developed, and the federal government through the NIH is both the performer of some and the funder of much biomedical research. Their conclusion is: "Lacking any particular way of determining the appropriate absolute level for research, one might as well select something of the order of magnitude that now exists—one that does provide the research environment essential to our institutions of higher education, that utilizes the talents of the majority of those with high levels of training and capacity in the field, and that provides the capacity for self-renewal in the education and training of young people."[7] Nevertheless, the authors realized that they had skirted two issues that had to be faced: allocation of resources within biomedical research and the weighing of alternatives between such research and other important federal programs.

A word or two about each of these two limitations. The responsibility for determining the proportions of the federal budget to be directed to basic research—more particularly basic biomedical research—and to specific areas of biomedical research, belonged to the Congress, whose final decision, while informed by the president's budget submissions, usually, as we noted earlier, exceeded these when it came to NIH appropriations. Economic theory would suggest that the preferred method of determining such allocations among government operating functions, basic research, and biomedical research should be guided by the opportunity costs of adding dollars to basic research or to biomedical research up to a point where the potential yield would exceed the benefits from alternative uses of such funds. However, economic theory provides little insight into congressional behavior or the decisions taken by the Appropriations committees and the final actions of the House and the Senate. These are governed primarily by the ease or difficulty in raising revenues relative to the strengths of various interest groups in securing new or enlarged appropriations for their priority programs and are influenced in no small measure by the prestige and skills of the key chairs of the key legislative committees.

In the middle 1970s the NIH engaged Selma Mushkin, a talented health economist, to undertake an in-depth analysis of the costs and benefits of biomedical research, the results of which were published in a book of 457 pages.[8] The NIH was responding to the less favorable attitudes and behavior of congressional Appropriations committees toward financing biomedical research. An increasing number of legislators were raising questions about the "returns" that the American people were getting from the large outlays for biomedical research. Mushkin, with the help of the NIH staff and outside collaborators, developed multiple sets of calculations that started at the turn of the century but concentrated on the period 1930–75. These calculations enabled her to compare the costs of research and the benefits as reflected in reduced mortality and morbidity. Mushkin, a sophisticated health economist, recognized that not all of the benefits could be ascribed to advances in research; many reflected gains in income, improvements in the environment, reduced stress, and still other determinants. And she made no effort to raise or answer the question of whether the social returns of research might have been greater had the Congress appropriated more funding for the National Science Foundation rather than the NIH. Nonetheless, she was willing to stand behind the following:

—"Net benefits, measured as benefits less the opportunity cost of research are between $115 and $137 billion over the period 1930–75 and from $227 to $402 billion over the period 1900–75."

—"A ratio of benefits to cost of one to one would not be disadvantageous to further investment."

—"In contrast, the benefits of biomedical research for the period 1930–75 are minimally four to six times the opportunity cost of the research and, for the period 1900–75, ten to sixteen times the opportunity cost of the research."

On the basis of these findings, Mushkin concluded: "Public policy on health research and development requires reassessment of decisions recently taken—reassessment that takes note of the favorable returns. The returns have been large by any investment standard: biomedical research has been worth its price."[9]

In 1985 the Committee on Science, Engineering, and Public Policy of the National Academy of Sciences established a subcommittee responsible for a workshop on the federal role in R & D, which explored two critical issues—measuring economic returns on federal investments in R & D and the appropriate principles for federal support of applied research. The principal conclusion was that "economic returns are not the explicit purpose of most federal investments in research and development—biomedical research is an example." The summary also noted that "economic analysis may not incorporate real benefits . . . overlooking gains accruing from maintaining the scientific enterprise, including research training."[10]

The subcommittee developed a table of federal funds for R & D by budget function for the period 1971–86.[11] It should be noted that in outlays for health, this approach leads to an undercount because the health care expenditures of the armed forces and veterans are subsumed under other budget functions. Over this sixteen-year span total outlays in current dollars increased from $15.5 billion to $58.3 billion, or slightly less than fourfold. However, because of the strong inflationary pressures that were present throughout most of this period, the increase measured in terms of constant dollars came to less than one-half.

Table 4.1 Federal Funds for R & D, 1971–1986 (In Constant $ Billions)

	1971	1975	1980	1986
Total	16.3	15.5	16.8	23.9
Defense	8.5	7.6	9.4	17.4
Health	1.4	1.8	2.1	2.1
Space	3.2	2.4	1.5	1.3

Source: National Academy of Sciences, National Academy of Engineering, Institute of Medicine, Committee on Science, Engineering, and Public Policy, *The Federal Role in Research and Development*, report of a workshop (Washington, D.C.: National Academy Press, 1986), 6–7.

Table 4.1 presents the changing trends among the totals and the three largest recipients of funds for selected years expressed in constant dollars.

Table 4.1 shows:

—The substantial stability in federal outlays during the 1970s.

—The acceleration in the 1980s, which was accounted for in its entirety by the larger appropriations for defense.

—The sharp declines in funding for space research and technology over the entire period.

—The absolute and relative increases in funding for health, amounting to a gain of 50 percent. Health moved from the third to the second position among the recipients.

The committee made brief comments about each of the major fields that received funding. About biomedicine it observed: "Among all the sciences, biomedicine delivers the most visible benefits of basic research. A breakthrough in understanding the nature of a disease can lead directly to treatment and to heartily appreciated benefits to individuals."[12]

In order to explore the economic returns to public R & D investments, the committee invited Jeffrey Harris, a physician and an economist at the Massachusetts Institute of Technology (MIT), to prepare a paper that would measure the returns on investment for biomedical research. Harris identified eight unresolved issues.[13]

—The synergistic interaction of basic and applied research makes it difficult to trace the path of innovation.

—Similarly, separating public from private R & D is difficult because of their mutual interdependence.

—Some biomedical innovations benefit from such diverse nonmedical R & D areas as sonar, lasers, fiber optics . . . computational science . . . radioisotope and nuclear chemistry. Identifying sources is complicated.

—Biomedical R & D is so international that foreign R & D must be considered a significant source of innovation.

—All improvements in health cannot be attributed to biomedical research; public health and life style changes may be important.

—Prolonging life may shift resources from the more productive young to the less productive elderly.

—Economics has made little advance in measuring the value of an improved quality of life.

—Many economic studies measure gains in productivity, but either the public's willingness to pay for medical innovations or the profits of private firms might be a more meaningful measure.

In connection with Harris's first observation, it is worth noting that the 42 percent that industry currently contributes to the more than $16 billion of total outlays for biomedical research is dependent on the federal government's funding about 90 percent of all basic research. Without the basic research, industry would have fewer leads to explore and exploit.

Concerning Harris's second point, we have noted the interdependence between the expenditures of the federal government for basic research and the outlays of industry for applied research and development. But the NIH subsumes within the term *private* the nonprofit sector, which includes universities and medical schools as well as research institutes and research hospitals. In chapter 2 we noted that this component of the research establishment performs a significant proportion of all biomedical research and a disproportionate share of basic research.

Harris's third observation is a reminder that, though specialization is the hallmark of scientific research, new ideas and new techniques are not discipline-bound, and biomedical research has borrowed much from (and presumptively contributed much to) the other natural sciences.

On the same topic as Harris's fourth point, we noted in chapter 3 that U.S. patents in the drug industry are approaching an equal distribution between U.S. and foreign origin and that U.S. pharmaceutical and related firms are increasing the proportion of their R & D effort undertaken abroad. To close the circle, we need add only that almost all of the leading European pharmaceutical firms have important subsidiaries in the United States, most of which engage in R & D activity.

In its concluding comments the committee presented additional observations about the inherent difficulties of applying a simple or, for that matter, even a complex cost-benefit approach to federal R & D. In relating federal R & D expenditures to GNP, the committee said, "Government's contribution is measured by its cost, not its value" Again, "improving the national health, for example, increases worker input as well as system output, resulting in no measurable net gain in productivity." Zvi Griliches of Harvard is quoted as saying that "a large portion of R & D funding goes to retrieving information and training people to take advantage of that information. Without R & D funding, our technical status would not simply stagnate, it would decline. This is an important economic benefit that is not measured."[14] The committee concluded that even if the methodology of economic modeling of R & D were greatly improved, it should be only one of many criteria for guiding R & D policy.

The burden of the foregoing analysis of the level of federal support for biomedical research and the correlative discussion about the return on the investment indicates that neither problem permits a singular answer. In a subsequent analysis, Griliches set forth in greater detail some of the difficulties in obtaining valid measures of the contribution of R & D to the nation's economy. The following are key excerpts from this article:

> The evidence of the economic impact of science and technology is all around us . . . Nevertheless, the quantitative scientific basis for these convictions is rather thin . . . The main difficulty lies in the unavailability of direct and relevant measures of the output of the R & D process and the resulting necessity of using indirect measures such as aggregate productivity growth, measures which may reflect the contribution of R & D investments imperfectly if at all.
>
> There are, roughly, three styles of research on the contribution of R & D to economic growth: historical case studies, analyses of inno-

vation counts and patent statistics, and econometric studies relating productivity to R & D and similar variables . . . On the whole, they tend to show rather high internal rates of return to private R & D expenditures and even higher social rates of return (on the order of 10–50% per year) . . .

Our national income accounts . . . do not reflect major components of the "product" of R & D and science and hence cannot serve as adequate measures of it . . . Or, taking another example, public research expenditures on health that lower the incidence of some disease: such a reduction of morbidity would, to a first approximation, raise both measured GNP and hours worked, leaving "productivity" (output per man hour) largely unchanged . . . Much, perhaps more than half of all U.S. R & D, is directed at outcomes where success is not reflected in the national output or productivity.[15]

The burden of Griliches' analysis is that conceptual and statistical limitations lead to results that tend to underestimate the contribution of R & D as currently measured to economic growth and national well-being.

At first glance it might appear that Mushkin, Harris, and Griliches approached the problem of estimating the costs and benefits of biomedical research quite differently. In point of fact, each was aware that the cost-benefit approach is at best imperfect and, in Griliches' view, tends to underestimate the full contribution of medical R & D. Mushkin was the most venturesome; she was willing to develop a range of estimates, emphasizing that even the lowest ratios suggested that the Congress would be justified in investing more of the taxpayers' money in medical R & D.

Moreover, the concentration of research in a relatively small number of favored institutions, which had been noted in the Bush report, has been altered only in part even after several decades of increased federal outlays for biomedical research. The report had noted that many medical schools, "because of inadequate financial support or lack of trained personnel . . . can contribute little to medical research. A great increase in the resources of the Nation would be achieved by stimulating research in these less favored schools."[16]

In 1967 the largest recipients of federal research money, arranged in descending order, were MIT, the University of Michigan, Columbia University, Harvard University, the University of Illinois, the University of California at Berkeley, Stanford University, the University of California at Los Angeles (UCLA), the University of Chicago, and the University of Wisconsin at Madison. Not a single university in the whole of the southern tier from the Atlantic to the Pacific was among the leaders. This would hold even if the list were extended to the top fifteen or twenty. It is not surprising, therefore, that many members of Congress, then as now, have been concerned by what they believe is a disproportionate concentration of federal funds flowing to a limited number of leading institutions, including the elite private institutions on the east coast.

In 1984 the top ten recipients included five east coast universities, Johns Hopkins, MIT, Columbia, Cornell, and Harvard, which together received 20 percent of the $5.6 billion of federal research money. Of the remaining five, four were located on the west coast: Stanford, the University of Washington (Seattle), UCLA, and the University of California at San Diego. Together with Wisconsin-Madison, these five received about 13 percent of all federal outlays for research. If we narrow the focus to the top ten NIH grantees for 1986, the list in descending order is: Johns Hopkins, the University of California at San Francisco, Yale, the University of Washington, Harvard, Stanford, the University of Pennsylvania, Columbia, UCLA, and the University of Minnesota.

These ten received $870 million of the $3.5 billion that the NIH made available to institutions of higher education. Although 1,608 institutions shared in the NIH grants, these ten received one-quarter of the total.

If we turn to the top ten recipients among medical schools, with few exceptions the list overlaps that of the top ten universities. Only Harvard, UCLA, and Minnesota are missing. They are replaced by Washington University (St. Louis), the Albert Einstein College of Medicine, and Duke University. Over the last decade medical schools have received just under one-half of all NIH funds. In 1986 the top ten alone received $691 million of a total NIH distribution to medical schools of $2.2 billion, or almost one out of every three dollars. Three of these ten are on the west coast. The University of California at San Francisco is first on the list of medical schools, with the University of Washington and Stanford in fourth and fifth place respectively. Only one medical school in the top ten, Washington University, is located between the two coasts. The others, all private—Yale, Columbia, Einstein, Pennsylvania, Johns Hopkins, and Duke—are located on the east coast between New Haven, Connecticut and Durham, North Carolina.

Despite the sensitivity of Bush and his advisory committee to the desirability of increasing the research potential of the regional medical schools, a concern that was shared by many in Congress and was given renewed expression by President Johnson when he talked of the desirability of creating new centers of excellence in the less developed regions of the country, the pattern of heavy concentration of research grants in a small number of institutions has not been significantly altered. The large federal funds flowing to the University of Washington reflect in considerable part the influence of a powerful senator, Warren Magnuson, the long-term chair of the Senate Appropriations Committee. Through his endeavors the University of Washington was able to join the top ten recipients of both university and medical school grants from the federal government.

The continuing concentration of biomedical research funds at a relatively small number of research institutions was more or less assured by the reliance of the NIH on the peer review system. The responsibility of the review panels was to judge the potential of the grant proposals, not to allocate funds for institution building. The money tended to flow to the researchers with the strongest research proposals, who for the most part were located at the major research centers.

In order not to overstate the long-term concentration phenomenon, it should be noted that, of the three west coast medical schools, only Stanford was included in the top ten (ranking tenth) in 1965–66, the other two and Duke not making the list. Einstein, which was established in 1955, ranked second because of the large amount in institutional support grants that it had received.

Four additional observations of the Bush report warrant at least brief mention because each of these issues has presented continuing challenges to those charged with responsibility for allocating federal funds.

The report warned that federal funds must not be available in such amounts as to encourage "mediocre work." In the formulation of fundamental principles governing the objectives of federal funding for medical research, the report stated: "A grave danger in any effort to accelerate discovery is the ease with which the quality of the work can be lowered by encouraging men to undertake research who are inadequately prepared or unfitted for the task. Mediocre research work in medicine is not only apt to be useless, but may prove dangerous by misleading medical practice and by fostering false hopes in the public. This danger must be guarded against by constantly encouraging confirmatory work or 'challenging investigations.' "[17]

During the era of large annual appropriations, a few informed observers emphasized anew the need for balance between competent researchers and the effective use of research funds. Since the end of the 1960s and early 1970s, however, the leaders of the research establishment have been more concerned about the shortfall in research dollars and the fact that many talented researchers' proposals are approved but not funded.

Though deliberate falsification of scientific data by unscrupulous investigators was not considered—a threat that was beyond imagining—there was a ready remedy against mediocre work that has applicability to the new menace, namely "constantly encouraging confirmatory work."

In the early and mid-1970s, of the 7,000–10,000 competing research proposals submitted annually to the NIH, almost 60 percent were approved. Thereafter there was a steep rise in the number of proposals reviewed, from 10,100 in 1976 to 19,100 in 1986, and of these from 70 to 90 percent were found eligible for funding. The most critical change relates to the decline in the ratio between the number of proposals found eligible and the number of grants actually awarded (see table 2.5). From a high of 61 percent found eligible and funded in 1975, the annual award rate dropped as low as 35 percent in 1982 and has risen only modestly since then. Table 4.2 shows the trend.

A combination of factors has been responsible for this ominous trend of falling ratios of projects actually funded to proposals found eligible for funding. The number of awards increased from around 2,700 in 1971 to more than double that number in 1986, when Congress increased the NIH's budget from its previous stabilization goal of 5,000 awards annually to over 6,000. The number of projects eligible for funding, however, had risen from 7,701 in 1975 to over 17,000 in fiscal year 1986, in part because the approval rate had risen from around 70 to about 90 percent. The conjunction of the research establishment's coming to maturity in the 1970s and the federal government's weakened budgetary

Table 4.2 Ratio of Funded to Eligible NIH Competing Research Projects, 1975–1986

Fiscal Year	Projects Reviewed	Projects Eligible for Funding	Projects Funded	Award Rate (%)
1975	10,893	7,701	4,663	61
1980	14,142	11,301	4,785	42
1982	16,989	14,477	5,027	35
1983	16,798	14,479	5,389	37
1985	18,675	16,763	6,247	37
1986	19,119	17,156	6,149	36

Source: U.S. Department of Health and Human Services, National Institutes of Health, *NIH Data Book* (Bethesda, Md., annual).

position provides the major explanation for the decline in the ratio of awards to approved proposals despite ameliorative actions taken by the NIH, the administration, and the Congress to increase the number of projects that could be funded.

In light of recent developments, perhaps the most interesting recommendation of the Bush report was its emphasis on providing medical students with the opportunity to pursue research training before beginning their clerkships by the provision of junior fellowships, "which would allow a medical student to interrupt his course, usually between the preclinical and clinical years, and to devote himself full-time to research for a year or two. The chances in this country for medical students to gain research experience prior to graduation are few, and as a result much research ability goes undiscovered."[18] The leadership of the research community has recently become disturbed by the declining proportion of MDs compared to PhDs who are competing successfully for first-time NIH grants. The leadership believes that if this trend continues, many investigators will not have the clinical knowledge and experience that would enable them to pursue many useful leads. Both basic and applied biomedical research could turn out to be less productive unless medically trained investigators play a larger role in the total research effort.

The fourth and final recommendation of the advisory committee to Bush also has a contemporary ring. "The Committee recognizes a great and urgent need for the expansion and renovation of medical school laboratories. However, our study has taken no account of this requirement, pertinent as it is to medical research, since a building program was considered outside of the scope of our assignment."[19]

On still another issue the prescience of the advisory committee is worth recapturing. One of the fundamental principles to which it directed attention was the potential danger of excessive domination of federal research dollars. "If the Government spends too much in medical research, other funds will be driven out and the Government will be the sole source of support." The committee went on to quote Senator Claude Pepper: "Government cannot, and must not, take the place of philanthropy and industry in the sponsorship of research."[20]

The foregoing has indicated the unusual insight of the members of the Bush committee in identifying the major issues on the nation's agenda involved in the future financing of biomedical research.

In 1986, Louis Harris and Associates interviewed on behalf of the Bristol-Myers Company 227 world-class scientists as part of a study "to examine priorities and primary areas of medical research in 'The Next Century.' " Skepticism about the results from sample interviews from the survey is surely in order when dealing with such complex matters as the future of biomedical research and its likely impact on reduction and eradication of disease. But the limitation of the survey to world-class research scientists justifies paying attention to the findings even though the results reveal a wide range of opinion.

The following are among the highlights of the report *Medicine in the Next Century*:[21]

—The new frontier for medical research is the fundamental understanding of cell mechanisms. While many recommend that basic research remain the top priority between now and the year 2000, they also see remarkable advances in prevention, diagnosis, and treatment of many diseases between now and then.

—The most important health problems in the West will be those stemming from an aging population.

—At the top of the list of priorities, cited by 29 percent of the scientists, is basic, fundamental research with heavy emphasis on cell biology and cancer.

—Scientists working in three of the specialty areas, cancer, biotechnology, and infectious diseases, predict there will be more than 1 million cases of AIDS in the United States by the year 2000. This is a median forecast. One-half of those interviewed were unwilling to make a forecast.

—Diseases most likely to be eliminated by the year 2000 are AIDS and measles, according to 19 and 17 percent of the scientists respectively.

—A majority (52 percent) see a cure for AIDS by the year 2010.

—Forty percent of the scientists consider the lack of adequate funds and financial support to be their chief frustration. Second on the list is government regulation (9 percent).

Turning to specific areas of investigation, we find the following expectations of scientists by field:

—Cancer: Leading researchers foresee an improved cure rate for cancer, with doctors curing two out of every three patients by the year 2000. A majority (60 percent) believe it will be possible to vaccinate people against certain types of cancer by the year 2000.

—Cardiovascular Disease: Researchers foresee elimination of most coronary bypass operations, which will be replaced by less invasive, catheter-based procedures or by clot-dissolving drugs requiring no surgery at all. Fully 90 percent of the researchers predict that better prevention will do more than either treatment or diagnosis to combat cardiovascular disease.

—The Central Nervous System: Fifty percent of the central nervous system researchers feel that traditional psychoanalytic therapy will be "somewhat unimportant" in the year 2000. Thirty-six percent believe it will be "not important at all."

—Infectious Diseases: The greatest improvement in the prevention of infectious diseases is anticipated for hepatitis (66 percent) and typhoid fever (49 percent). By contrast, 57 percent see no progress in preventing colds.

—Nutrition: The fundamental question in nutritional research will be metabolism and its regulation—how nutrients are dealt with at the cellular level. In the clinical area, 53 percent say doctors will advise patients to eat fiber-containing foods to help prevent cancer, and 63 percent say doctors will advise patients to limit consumption of cholesterol in the interest of preventing heart disease.

—Biotechnology: The development of genetically engineered vaccines is seen as the most promising area of research. Biotechnology researchers see much or some improvement in the prevention or treatment of AIDS (72 percent), hepatitis (81 percent), and malaria (72 percent) from the products of biotechnology. However, among the 227 scientists surveyed, a larger number (26 percent) singled out cancer more than any other disease as likely to benefit from biotechnology.

—Medical Implants: The most important and primary area of research for medical implants lies in the development of non-immunogenic materials. Scientists are particularly optimistic about implants for the treatment of arthritis (91 percent), diabetes (87 percent), hormonal defects (87 percent), deafness (83 percent), and cardiovascular disease (82 percent). Artificial knees, hips, skin, and blood are also expected to be more widely used.

There are several ways to read this report. First, it is important to remember that the year 2000 is only 12 years away, a short period in terms of the time usually required for turning research into treatment and cure. Second, it is worth observing that the researchers are cautious when it comes to finding answers to three of the most serious health challenges that we face, cures for or prevention of AIDS, cancer, and cardiovascular disease. On the other hand, they see many areas in which significant progress is likely to occur, including better outcomes for patients afflicted with cancer or heart disease. On balance, they are cautious about the role of preventive and therapeutic advances in cancer, and they do not share the pessimism of some critics of the National Cancer Institute.

Most important, within the context of our analysis, their chief concern is the shortage of funds for basic research because they see the prospect of major gains from intensified exploration of cell biology.

What lessons can be extracted from the last four decades of large increases in national funding for biomedical research that might better inform the discussion of how many dollars are enough?

The data and analyses we have reviewed point to mixed lessons.

—Funding should be sufficient to maintain the biomedical research establishment at a level that enables it to make productive use of its skilled investigators and allows for the renewal of both its physical plant and equipment and its human resources.

—Wide fluctuations in financing should be avoided since they place the research infrastructure under stress, with more money than capable investigators available during good times and insufficient funds to maintain competent workers when resources are constrained.

—There is no simple or even complex way of using economic models to determine the cost-benefit relationships of different levels of research funding. The value of output of biomedical research cannot be measured quantitatively. One reasonable prescription is that a modern society that does not support a sizable research infrastructure will not remain in the forefront of the global economy for long.

—The federal government must remain the principal funder of basic research. A sound decision was made when Congress looked to the universities and their medical schools to carry out most of the basic research that is federally funded.

—There is nothing in the data or analysis to indicate that the United States is directing too much of its annual income to the support of biomedical research. The weight of the evidence suggests that incremental additions might be in order.

—The National Science Foundation has accumulated evidence that as a result of constrained federal support since the early and mid-1970s, the research infrastructure of universities and medical schools needs to be strengthened by modernization of facilities, and there is considerable evidence pointing to the need for additional funding for research training of clinical investigators and for the support of large interdisciplinary efforts.

—It does not seem practical or even desirable in the face of the present and prospective federal deficit for the nation to pursue an aggressive funding policy to establish a number of new centers of excellence in biomedical research. The cost would be high and the redistribution of scarce resources could be dysfunctional.

—Since the federal budget is likely to remain unbalanced for many years to come and in fact might become even more unbalanced in the event of a severe and/or prolonged recession, it is fortunate that the United States has continued to rely on multiple sources of funding for biomedical research. In 1987 industry's share, largely concentrated in applied research and development, was about 42 percent of the total, while the federal government's share, which came to about 47 percent of the total, provided almost all of the funding for basic research.

—At this point in the nation's development, it is desirable to look more closely at the role of philanthropy, whose share has steadily declined in the post–World War II era, but which nonetheless may have the potential of making a considerably larger contribution both through strengthening the infrastructure of biomedical research and through funding critical areas neglected by other funders.

5 · The Philanthropic Dimension

A retrospective view is essential to an analysis of the present situation and the prospects for the role of philanthropy in biomedical research. As we indicated earlier, on the eve of World War II, philanthropy was second only to industry as a source of funds for biomedical research, accounting for $17 million of a total national outlay of $45 million, or roughly 38 percent of the total.

Although in absolute terms the current dollar contribution from private nonprofit sources to biomedical research increased sixfold between 1950 and 1987, and even in constant dollars at half that rate, at least, its relative share never returned to the high water mark of 1940. There was a steady decline to 22 percent in 1950 and to 14 percent a decade later and finally a stabilization at about 4 percent from 1981 to the present, with a total projected figure for 1987 of about $700 million (see table 2.2). Though this last figure is probably an understatement, philanthropy accounted for only a small share of the total funds available for biomedical research in 1987.

Refinement of these figures is less important than arriving at a broader understanding of the trends in philanthropy at large, with special attention to the health sector and specifically to medical research. It is a reasonable presumption that the potential of philanthropy to make a greater contribution to medical research will depend in no small measure on trends in total philanthropic giving, particularly donations to the health sector.

The data that follow are drawn in large part from *Giving USA: Estimates of Philanthropic Giving in 1986 and the Trends They Show.*[1] Several caveats are in order about data involving philanthropy. There is no established data collecting system for the whole of philanthropy. The American Association of Fund-Raising Counsel, Inc. (AAFRC) is recognized to be the best source, and its estimates are accepted as the official figures on philanthropy in the *Statistical Abstract of the United States.*[2] However, the AAFRC data relating to "giving by individuals," by far the largest component, are based on an analysis of income tax returns. Prior to the 1986 tax law reform, taxpayers could readily exaggerate the amount of their donations; hence the reported figures may be overstated to a significant degree. But there is no reason to believe that the extent of this bias varies from year to year. However uncertain the base, the trend data would seem to have substantial validity.

Other data collected by AAFRC, usually in association with various philanthropic organizations, are based on representative samples. The data that follow are the best available, and we believe that although they are second-order derivations, they are sufficiently robust to support the ensuing analysis.

It is estimated that in 1986 Americans gave $87.2 billion to a cross-section of the nation's more than 350,000 gift-supported organizations and agencies. The total for 1986 represented an increase of 9.4 percent over 1985, well above the inflation rate. From 1955 to 1986 total giving rose from $7.7 billion to $87.22, an elevenfold increase. Even in constant dollars there was a tripling of donations. Between 1960 and 1980 gifts doubled every decade, so that, if this trend continues, by 1990 the total will come to at least $100 billion in current dollars.

From 1970 to 1972 philanthropic giving amounted on average to a little over 2 percent of the GNP, but it declined thereafter to a low of 1.8 percent in 1979. Since then there has been a fairly steady recovery, so that by 1986 the 1972 level had almost been reestablished.

Donors

There are four major groups of donors—individuals, bequests, foundations, and corporations (including corporate foundations) (table 5.1 and fig. 5.1). Individual gifts have always dominated the total, contributing on average four out of every five dollars since 1955. When bequests are added together with individual gifts, the

Table 5.1 Donors and Recipients of Philanthropic Giving, 1986

	Percentage	$ billion
Donors		
Individuals	82.2	71.72
Bequests	6.7	5.83
Foundations	5.9	5.17
Corporations	5.2	4.50
Total	100.0	$87.22
Recipients		
Religion	46.9	40.9
Education	14.6	12.73
Health	14.0	12.26
Human Services	10.5	9.13
Arts and Culture	6.7	5.83
Public/Society	2.7	2.38
Other	4.6	3.99
Total	100.0	$87.22

Source: American Association for Fund-Raising Counsel, Trust for Philanthropy, *Giving USA: Estimates of Philanthropic Giving in 1986 and the Trends They Show,* 32d annual issue (New York, 1987).

combined totals account for nine of every ten dollars. Of total giving of $87.2 billion in 1986, individual gifts came to $71.7 billion, bequests to $5.8 billion, together accounting for 89 percent. Foundation giving of $5.2 billion contributed almost 6 percent, while corporations gifts of $4.5 billion provided a little over 5 percent.

Using 1980 as a base, we find that corporations had increased their giving in 1986 by 90 percent; giving by foundations rose by 83 percent; bequests increased by 104 percent; and individual giving rose by 78 percent. It is probably premature to read too much into this recent trend in light of the cautious attitudes of many informed persons with regard to the future contributions of U.S. corporations (particularly if the economy should experience a recession) and the sensitivity of foundation giving to the changing values of securities holdings. Despite these cautionary notes, there are several factors favorable to the growth of nonindividual gifts.

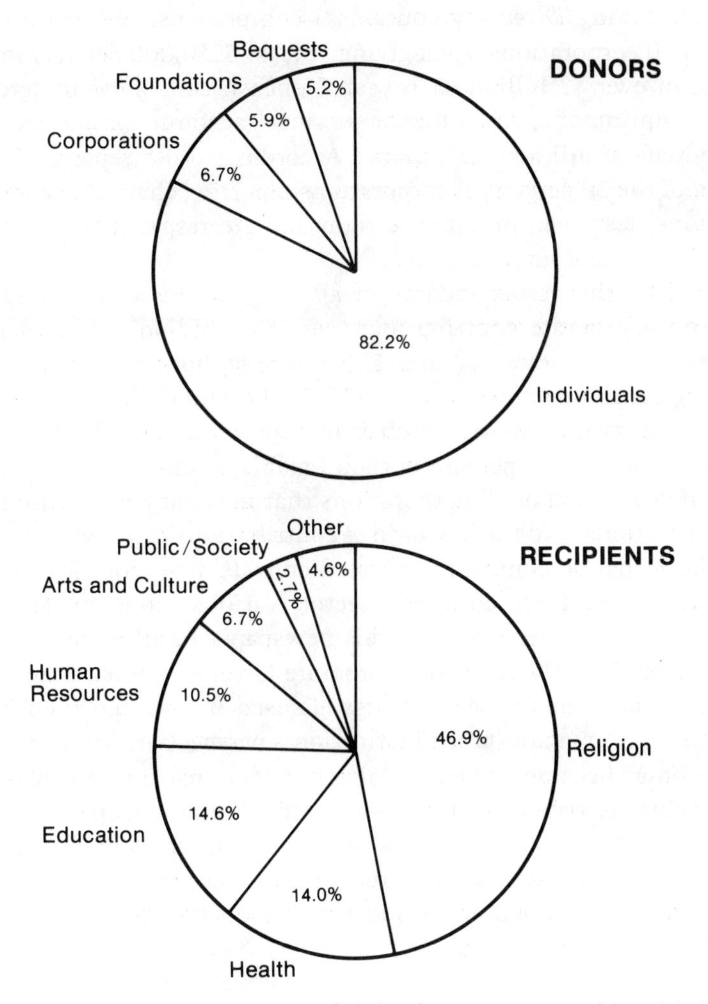

Figure 5.1 Donors and Recipients of Philanthropic Giving, 1986
Source: Table 5.1.

Corporations

Corporate giving refers to direct giving by corporations not channeled through a charitable foundation. According to the Taft Group, a provider of professional services to nonprofit institutions, more than one-half of all major corporations, including five of the ten largest, give directly from pretax profits. The *Taft Corporate Giving Directory* contains a comprehensive directory of over 570 corporations, each giving at least $250,000 per year for a total of over $2 billion each year. Noncash contributions (products, equipment, and in-kind services) account for additional hundreds of millions of dollars.[3] According to IRS reports, however, of the 30 percent of corporations reporting charitable contributions, less than one in one thousand are responsible for one-half of total corporate giving.[4]

In 1986 the pretax income of all corporations came to $235 billion. Corporate contributions were $4.5 billion, just under 2 percent of corporate income. This figure is, however, double the average gift to income ratio of 1976–79. In light of the continuing favorable tax provisions, which enable corporations to deduct contributions up to 10 percent of their taxable income, the relatively small proportion of all corporations that make any philanthropic contributions, and the low ratio of contributions to pretax income of those that do contribute, there is considerable scope for larger donations from the corporate sector. Various economic factors may, of course, intervene, as this newspaper headline indicates: "Mergers Thin the Ranks of Corporate Givers." "When Standard Brands and Nabisco became first Nabisco Brands and then RJR Nabisco, from a non-profit institution's perspective, three potential donors became one potential donor. If an institution had been receiving contributions from two, perhaps three companies that merged into one, it's unlikely that the nonprofit would receive one gift equal in size to the three formerly received."[5] The fear of the adverse effect of mergers and acquisitions may be exaggerated, but it cannot be ignored.

Foundations

The outlook for increased foundation giving is uncertain since it is contingent largely upon the grant-making decisions of the private foundations, especially those with assets above $10 million, whose combined grants amounted to $5.2 billion, or over 60 percent of total foundation giving, in 1986. In the health area there are two major types of foundation: private foundations and operating foundations, also known as voluntary health agencies, which are public charities primarily supported by the general public, such as the American Cancer Society.

The Independent Sector, a coalition of over 650 national voluntary organizations, foundations, and corporation contribution programs, has launched a five-year plan called "Daring Goals for a Caring Society: A Blueprint for Substantial Growth in Giving and Volunteering in America," to double charitable giving and volunteering by 1991. The goal is to increase the $80 billion contributed in 1985 to $160 billion dollars in 1991. Even if this ambitious program were to fall short of its goal, the leaders of the Independent Sector clearly anticipate that an increased total will be available for distribution in 1991.

Recipients

The recently revised category schema in *Giving USA* distinguishes among seven areas as the major recipients of philanthropy: religion, education, health, social services, arts and humanities, civic and public benefit, and "other."[1]

Religion has long commanded the largest proportion of philanthropic giving; in 1986 its share came to slightly under one-half (46.9 percent). This share has increased by several percentage points since 1970 and even since 1980.

Education and health are the next two major recipients, accounting in 1986 for 14.6 percent and 14.1 percent respectively. In 1985 the relative positions of the two were reversed; health was in second position, just slightly ahead of education. It should be noted that colleges and universities receive the largest share of all the money contributed to education, accounting in the academic year 1985–86 for 68 percent of all gifts to education. Since most of the nation's leading research universities operate medical schools and many of them own their teaching hospitals, it is often difficult to know how gifts and endowment income are divided between the university proper and its medical school. Moreover, the relationship between the two in the fund-raising arena is complicated by the different practices of universities, some engaging in a single large campaign while others embark on separate or coordinated campaigns. We do know, however, that there are important spillover effects, some favoring one, and some favoring the other.

Another facet of the relationship between the university proper and its medical center relates to the uses to which gifts to higher educational institutions are directed. In 1985–86, of the total of $7.4 billion contributions to education, a little less than one-half ($3.4 billion) was for capital purposes. An inspection of the "Large Gifts to Education" listed in *Giving USA* indicates that seven gifts of $50 million or more went to major universities and to research institutions, most of which had outstanding medical schools or engaged in biological and medical research. They included Stanford, Washington University (St. Louis), the University of Miami, the California Institute of Technology, the Scripps Research Clinic, and the Menninger Foundation. The combined total of these seven largest gifts to higher education amounted to $670 million.

Though there is no firm basis for estimating how much of this sizable sum was directed to biomedical research, it is reasonable to assume that some part, possibly a significant part, went toward capital construction and/or equipment of laboratories and the strengthening of faculty engaged in biomedical research.

An inspection of the list of gifts between $1 million and $50 million reveals that a number had been directed specifically to medical centers or medical schools and that many more went to universities with a strong track record in the sciences and medicine. In sum, a considerable portion of the $7.4 billion contributed to higher education certainly became available for biomedical research.

Giving to Health

In 1986 philanthropy contributed $12.2 billion directly to the nation's hospitals, health services, and medical research, a figure within the range of the $14.4 billion total contributed during the same year by the federal government, industry, and private nonprofit organizations to the support of biomedical research.[6]

In 1970 philanthropic giving for health amounted to $3.4 billion, and a decade later the figure had doubled to $6.7 billion, but most of this increase reflected inflation. In light of the reduction in the rate of inflation after 1982, the increase from $9.2 billion in 1983 to $12.2 billion in 1985 is impressive, amounting to $3 billion, or one-third, in this brief period.

The information available from AAFRC, as well as from supplementary sources, does not permit a definitive analysis of the sources of the increased giving or the purposes for which the philanthropic funds were used. However, it is possible to piece together a composite picture that provides perspective on these flows of funds and their disposition.

The 1986 figures for all philanthropic giving trace 82 percent to individual gifts and just under 7 percent to bequests. According to the AAFRC staff, modest adjustments of these ratios are required with regard to the health sector: individual gifts accounted for about 80 percent of the total and bequests about 10 percent for a total of 90 percent from these sources.

Giving USA estimates that in 1986 about 29 percent of all corporate gifts and about 22 percent of all foundation gifts went to the health category. It would seem that of the total giving for health of $12.2 billion, about 90 percent, or $11 billion, originated in individual gifts and bequests and the remaining 10 percent or $1.2 billion came from corporations and foundations. The same source provides some leads on the disposition of philanthropic funds within the health area.

Information was furnished by the National Association for Hospital Development about fund raising by 1,300 of the nation's 7,000 acute care hospitals that it surveyed. Included in the survey were 234 medical centers, which presumably include most or all of the principal teaching affiliates of the nation's 128 medical schools and other large teaching hospitals.[7]

The surveyed hospitals reported that they had raised $1.3 billion in cash gifts in 1986. In addition they obtained $665 million in pledges and planned gifts. These gifts represented donations from 2.2 million individuals.

The following groups contributed to the sampled hospitals an average of about $200 million each: corporations, foundations, and members of the hospital family (trustees, medical and other staff, employees).

More than one-quarter of the hospitals reported that they were involved in a capital campaign (presumably the high pledge figure noted above was related to this effort) and over two-fifths planned to establish a foundation. According to the summary by the National Association for Hospital Development, the hospitals used their donated funds for, in descending order, construction and renovation, equipment, general operations, endowment, research and teaching, and equity or financing.

Clearly, hospitals and other health care institutions are the primary instrumentalities through which philanthropy seeks to support the health sector. Governmental data suggest that the philanthropic contribution to hospital care will be in the $2.5 billion range in 1987; over $5 billion will be donated to pay for personal health care services.

The major operating foundations or voluntary health agencies provide a second major conduit for donations to health. The six largest, each with $79 million or more in annual contributions, are, in descending order, the American Cancer Society, the American Heart Association, the March of Dimes–Birth Defects Foundation, the Muscular Dystrophy Association, the National Easter Seal Society, and the American Lung Association. The fifteen major foundations had total revenues of about $700 million in fiscal year 1985, of which $158 million was spent on biomedical research.[8]

According to a survey undertaken by AAFRC, these agencies revealed a current volunteer strength in excess of 15.3 million persons; each of the four largest—the American Cancer Society, the American Heart Association, the Muscular Dystrophy Association, and United Cerebral Palsy—reported a total of between 2 and 2.5 million volunteers. The largest number of these volunteers are active in fundraising, but sizable numbers, between 100,000 and 300,000 per agency, contribute other forms of service. It should be noted that the dollar value of formal volunteering is estimated at $110 billion a year, a figure 30 percent above the total philanthropic dollars that are raised. The last survey, in 1985, revealed a total of 89 million volunteers, with an average weekly commitment of 3.5 hours per person.

It is likely that the $156 million that these agencies received in 1986 from bequests, which amounted to 16 percent of their total contributions, was in part a reflection of the large number of volunteers they had been able to engage. The two largest agencies, the American Cancer Society and the American Heart Association, were the beneficiaries of $71 million and $40 million respectively in bequests.

Thus far we have identified two principal objectives of philanthropic giving in the health area: payment for personal health care services by hospitals and other institutions and the many functions supported or performed by the voluntary health agencies, among them patient care services, public education, research, and professional training.

The AAFRC lists thirty large gifts in the category of health in 1986, the first five of which totaled over $100 million. Sixteen of these gifts were distributed to universities and medical centers, four to hospitals, five to research centers, and five for public health purposes. This list suggests that large donors are concerned less with defraying expenses incurred by patient care and more with strengthening the health care infrastructure, including medical schools and biomedical research.

In 1975, Robert Blendon wrote "The Changing Role of Private Philanthropy in Health Affairs," in which article he noted the following changes in that role between the pre- and post-World War II periods:[9]

—In the prewar era philanthropy supported seven main kinds of activities: medical research, medical and public health education, development of community hospitals, the medical needs of the poor and near-poor, emergency medical relief, programs to improve the health of minority Americans, and technical and financial assistance to the developing nations.

—In the postwar era, because of the increasing dominance of federal financing for health, philanthropy has dedicated its health funds to activities in four areas: venture capital for the formulation of new projects and ideas; funding for projects that go beyond the limits of current governmental funding; grants that serve as "critical glue" to underwrite losses of hospitals and clinics that serve low-income and poor patients; and support of community-supervised out-of-hospital medical care programs.

Blendon distinguished between foundations that made primarily "investment goods" types of grant and "consumption goods" awards. According to his calculations, over half of every foundation dollar is directed to programs and demonstrations aimed at improving the delivery of health care services and the training of personnel; about one-quarter is directed to the construction of facilities and one-tenth is directed to medical research. The remainder is used for financing health services and other expenditures. He placed strong emphasis on the potential impact of the investment of foundation funds in efforts to assure that public sector health activities are conducted effectively and in educating the public about health care issues.

This discussion of the several dimensions of philanthropy can be amplified by the findings of a recently released special report entitled *Health Giving Patterns of Philanthropic Foundations 1975, 1980, and 1983.*[10] As the title indicates, this study, directed by Betty L. Dooley at the Center for Health Policy Studies at the Georgetown University School of Medicine, focuses on foundations to the exclusion of other sources of philanthropic giving. We will concentrate on the data for 1983, a year in which national health expenditures amounted to $355 billion. (In 1987 the total had risen to $497 billion, or by some 40 percent.)

Figures presented for 1983 are these: philanthropy (other than private and community grant-making foundations) $8.7 billion; foundations, $712 million; other (including industrial in-plant health services and privately financed construction), $1.5 billion. The combined total of these three categories comes to almost $10.9 billion, or 3.1 percent of national health expenditures. Foundations contributed only $1 toward health expenditures compared to $12 contributed by other sources of philanthropy. (Figures for neither the Markey Charitable Trust nor the Howard Hughes Medical Institute, which is technically not a foundation, are included.)

With regard to the uses to which foundation funds were directed, the largest category was research (including health services research), which amounted to 35 percent of the $712 million total, followed closely by current services (grants for direct medical care and general operating support), which accounted for 31 percent. Construction and equipment accounted for 21 percent, and education and training of health professionals for 13 percent. Over the nine-year span (1975–83), the most striking changes were the relative decline in spending for construction and equipment from 40 to 21 percent and the increases of around ten percentage points for both current services and research. When the inflationary factor is removed, total foundation giving for health over this period declined by 12 percent, although grants for biomedical research increased about 10 percent.

The general trends in foundation giving for health are summarized as follows: the erosion of foundations' assets as a consequence of the prolonged period of inflation and a weak stock market led them to decrease their giving for health while they sought to redirect their giving to meet new demands on them. Within the health area they cut back on support for construction (as a result of excess bed capacity) and on training of health professionals because of the emerging surplus of physicians; they increased their outlays for health services research in the hope and expectation of contributing to the urgent national need to improve the utilization of the health system's total resources.

This is how the author appraised the biomedical research arena: "It is expected that both the share and value of biomedical research will increase in the near future as several foundations have decided to fund research on specific diseases or simply basic research. The primary example is the Lucille P. Markey Foundation which will be funding basic biomedical research until 1997 at the extraordinarily high level of $40 million or more per year. In addition the millions of dollars flowing from the unique Hughes Medical Institute . . . cannot be ignored in assessing the patterns of future support for this activity."[11]

Another analysis, the Pew Charitable Trusts report, *U.S. Funding for Biomedical Research* (1987), indicates that 364 of the 4,000 largest private U.S. foundations offered some form of support for biomedical research in fiscal year 1985. Of these, 19 with combined assets of over $9 billion are analyzed in some detail. They include the John D. and Catherine T. MacArthur Foundation, the Pew Charitable Trusts, the Rockefeller Foundation, the Alfred P. Sloan Foundation, the Lucille P. Markey Charitable Trust, the Henry J. Kaiser Family Foundation, the Edna McConnell Clark Foundation, and other well known foundations. The Howard Hughes Medical Institute is analyzed separately. Twenty percent of all grant money, over $80 million, was allocated for biomedical grants.[12]

This broad look at the role of philanthropy in U.S. society has placed particular emphasis on the part it plays in the funding of health, specifically biomedical research. Despite the absence of a firm statistical base, it is possible to piece together from a number of discrete sources the broad outlines of the philanthropic dimension.

—Total annual contributions to philanthropy in the United States approached $90 billion in 1986, and many among the leadership believe that if the economy does not falter, giving may reach $160 billion by 1991.

—Over the recent period, health and education have been jockeying for second place behind religion, the dominant beneficiary, which continues to command slightly less than one-half of all donations from all sources. Health and hospitals currently receive about one of every seven dollars disbursed by philanthropy.

—The major contributions to philanthropy are made overwhelmingly by individuals, followed far behind by bequests, corporations, and foundations.

—A rough calculation suggests that perhaps as much as $2.5–3 billion is contributed to hospitals and that in addition, more than $2 billion is given to a variety of disease- and disability-oriented national health agencies that provide services to patients and engage in broad public education. These agencies also spend some of their funds on research and the training of professionals.

—The data do not permit identification of any large source of philanthropic funding intended specifically for biomedical research other than the contributions of foundations, which in 1983 spent $133 million for this purpose.

—*Giving USA, 1986* showed combined philanthropic outlays for hospitals and national health agencies of $4.5 billion. The governmental data in the *Statistical Abstract, 1987* show philanthropic support for personal health care services amounting to $4.9 billion for 1985. In addition, the governmental data show $5.5 billion for private construction of facilities and $400 million for research, both for the year 1985. The combined governmental data indicate a total philanthropic (private) outlay of $10.8 billion. Data found in *Giving USA* on philanthropic contributions for health in 1985 show a total of $11.3 billion, virtually the same total as that estimated by the Health Care Financing Administration. But our concern is less with pointing to the conformity among gross totals and more with the significant spillover effects of the large outlays for construction, part of which help to strengthen the biomedical research infrastructure.

6 · Academic Health Centers

Background

Passing reference has been made to the contributions of the AHCs to biomedical research. The highlights are recapitulated below to set the background for assessing the potential of philanthropy to make a greater contribution to this critical resource.

—The leading medical schools were the principal locale for the modest amount of basic and clinical research in medicine that was carried on in the United States prior to World War II.

—When the government and the medical leadership agreed that the federal government should assume a broader responsibility in the post–World War II era for financing biomedical research, they quickly decided that the site of such research should continue to be the medical schools. This speedy consensus was a consequence of the lack of real competitors to medical schools in offering a viable alternative; further, the leadership agreed that important gains could be achieved by keeping research and professional education and training within the same environment.

—There was an understanding among the interested parties—the medical schools, the federal government, and the American Medical Association—that because of the interlocking relationships among the education, research, and patient care conducted at AHCs, part of the overhead on federal research funding could be used by the medical centers to ease their increasingly strained educational budgets. Before long, part or all of the salaries for the increased research faculty was charged against federal research grants.

—The commingling of research and other funds did not end with overhead and faculty salaries. With the establishment of Medicare and Medicaid in 1965, a new large source of federal funding became available to the AHCs via reimbursement for patient care. Since at that time Medicare used a cost-reimbursement approach in paying hospitals for treating Medicare patients, the large centers that combined teaching, research and patient care were able to charge much of their clinical research to patient reimbursement and were also able to use some part of the physician reimbursement funds for the support of their research programs. After the prospective payment system was put in place in 1983, Medicare continued to pay large teaching hospitals at a special rate to compensate for their involvement in graduate medical education and in the treatment of more seriously ill patients.[1]

—There is more to the complex sources of federal funding of the AHCs. The NIH, for example, financed various types of grants to centers, which provided important support for training research personnel. In the period from 1963 to 1973, sizable federal funds were made available for construction of health facilities (including research facilities), capitation, and related purposes geared to larger student enrollments and special aid for low-income and minority students. These special educational support funds did not wind down until the end of the 1970s, and thereafter only small sums were appropriated.

—The conventional wisdom about the post–World War II experience in the funding of biomedical research underscores the following propositions, particularly with respect to the AHCs:

- The federal government, largely through the NIH, became the dominant source of funds for research at the AHCs, and, in the years of accelerating appropriations (mid-1960s), federal funds accounted for at least one-half of the total revenues of the leading research-oriented medical centers.
- Though it is impossible to trace directly the effect of this increased federal funding of biomedical research on philanthropic giving, it is true that over the years philanthropy accounted for a drastically reduced share of the enlarged total.

- However, this gross comparison may hide almost as much as it discloses. We called attention in chapter 5 to the sizable sums that philanthropy has continued to direct toward the construction of health care and research facilities, a sum much greater than its direct grants for research.
- Moreover, the current governmental reporting systems do not include contributions to the financing of biomedical research that derive from the endowment income of medical schools which covers a sizable proportion of the salaries and office expenses of many professors and administrators.
- With the current reporting system it is impossible to identify the percentage of practice income, currently the single largest component of medical school income, that is used directly or indirectly for the support of biomedical research.
- Another development concerns the recently energized activities of leading state university medical schools to attract philanthropic funds for both capital and operating purposes.
- In 1984–85 federal funding of $2.4 billion from all sources, dominated by funding for biomedical research of over $2 billion, accounted for 25 percent of the total revenues of medical schools, a far lower percentage than in the peak years. Because the preponderance of the research funds went to a relatively small number of major research-oriented AHCs, the proportion of federal funding in these institutions was considerably higher.[2]

A Survey of Major Centers of Biomedical Research

The foregoing suggests that, for a clearer view of the role of philanthropy in biomedical research, it would be desirable, even necessary, to survey both a group of leading AHCs and a group of large teaching hospitals that are not the principal affiliates of medical schools but are engaged in biomedical research.

The survey was initiated in 1986, with an assurance of anonymity. Summary financial data were requested, and, in the case of the AHCs, the opinions of the chancellor or vice president for health affairs, the dean of the medical school, or the director of the university hospital were elicited about the prospects for additional funding by philanthropy.

The survey instrument differentiated among government; large public foundations; and private foundations, individual donors, and bequests as sources of funding for biomedical research.

Academic Health Centers

Ten AHCs were selected from among different regions of the country, including both nonprofit institutions and state universities. There were two common characteristics: each was a major center for biomedical research, and the director of Conservation of Human Resources had a sufficiently close personal relationship with the chief administrators to anticipate that they would all respond.

Nine of the ten respondents gave quantitative information. Their replies revealed that total grants, contracts, and gifts for biomedical research from *all* sources varied from an annual low of $34 million to a high of $117 million, with an average of around $70 million. These figures include support for both operating and capital purposes, restricted and unrestricted gifts, the endowment of professorships, and all other forms of support for biomedical R & D.

We requested information for each of three years, 1983, 1984, and 1985. We found that, on average, the total level of support had increased over this period by 27 percent.

There was substantial variation in the amount of funds received from private foundations and individual donors as a percentage of all nongovernmental grants and contracts received. In two AHCs this source accounted for 50–60 percent; in another two, for 22–32 percent; in yet another two, for 10 and 14 percent respectively; and in three, for less than 5 percent.

A more critical consideration of philanthropic giving as a percentage of *all* grants, contracts, and gifts reveals that in the three institutions with the largest philanthropic donations, private foundations and individual donors contributed between 9 and 16 percent of all biomedical research funds. In the next two, the percentages were much lower, 3.5–4.7 percent, and in the remainder, even lower.

Over the three-year period 1983–85, the proportion of private philanthropy as a percentage of total nongovernmental support increased. At one AHC, this proportion rose from about 33 percent to 50 percent of all biomedical research funds. In the other cases the gain was more modest, from 3 to 10 percentage points.

More revealing than the foregoing were the replies we received to each of three questions that we put to the administrators.

Question 1
Does your recent experience lead you to assess the potential for private philanthropy to be substantial or modest?

Replies
1. Our experience here has been that the potential for private philanthropy is substantial.

2. My recent experience leads me to assess the potential for private philanthropy to be substantial at———. This institution is still relatively unknown among wealthy individuals. Those who are familiar with———often have the misconception that the state of———provides the majority of our revenues. ———'s Development Office has been in operation for only three years. Even with these limitations, ——— raised nearly $36 million last year, which places it in the top forty universities in the country for fund raising.

My only reservations concerning ———'s philanthropic potential are related to the new tax laws.

3. I think private philanthropy has been increasing its support very nicely. One great concern to me is whether the new tax law (if enacted) will permit this trend to continue in the long-range future.

4. Since the ——— Medical School is about to launch a major Capital Campaign, you will understand that I believe that the potential for private philanthropy in support of biomedical research is substantial. On the other hand, the competition for such funds is intense.

5. I believe the potential for private philanthropy is substantial. While it can never replace NIH and NSF [National Science Foundation] funding, certainly it can add significantly. I can give four examples out of my own experience in the last three years—Dean ——— could give much more insight. These gifts for pain treatment, alcoholism, cancer treatment, and inflammatory bowel disease have totalled $12.5 million from four donors; some of [these gifts] will function as endowments, some as seed money, and some for bricks and mortar. The trick is to find people interested in specific projects (most often grateful patients and families), have outstanding people to sell, and work at it. The institutions most likely to be successful are those [that] lead from strength in research already.

Donors (particularly Foundations) are becoming more sophisticated in identifying areas of need, i.e., where federal funds are inadequate. The Lucille P. Markey Charitable Trust is an excellent example of such a donor. Institutions which are able to articulate these unmet needs to private donors are increasingly successful. The tax reform legislation has caused some concern for this trend, though my reading of the provisions suggests that the impact will be minimal on most wealthy donors.

6. My impression is that the potential of private philanthropy is substantial. A great deal of money is being made by contemporary entrepreneurs in a whole spectrum of high tech and service markets. I am sure they have native philanthropic instincts but I believe they can be cultivated over time. It is human to want "status" and giving significant gifts/grants is one way to achieve that end.

Most of us in institutions like ours are working to educate those who have recently acquired great wealth to the importance of philanthropy. In view of the general economy and the federal attitude towards social programs, we have no alternative but to succeed or lose the progress of the past thirty years.

7. Our recent experience is that the potential for individual donor support for biomedical research is substantial. The key is to explain the importance of such an investment and the relationship of basic research to improved health. It is difficult because the payoffs are uncertain and research is costly and time-consuming. But if the message is conveyed properly and the donor is properly cultivated, then I believe that the funding of research is an attractive philanthropic opportunity. Philanthropists are interested in humanitarian concerns, and research is one such avenue.

As for foundation support, we have not had too much success in obtaining major research grants. It seems that, although large sums are available, the grants are awarded to a handful of institutions. And it's tough to break into the club.

8. We are engaged in a capital campaign to raise $125 million in private funding for the ——— School of Medicine, one quarter of which will support programs and research. We underestimated the resourcefulness of our faculty in raising private research funds, so we have already exceeded our program and research objectives. Thus, my answers are based on recent experience.

Prior to the campaign, the School's search for private funding was not aggressive, and the results reflected it. Today, with $88 million pledged toward the total campaign goal, we are committed to a long-term development program which will build upon the success of these more ambitious efforts.

For the foreseeable future, private research funding will equal only a fraction of the amount ——— received from NIH; ——— ranks very high among medical schools receiving NIH funding. However, our endowment of $85 million is modest compared with other leading schools, so we have chosen to devote most of our private fund-raising efforts toward increasing our endowment, and expanding and renovating our buildings.

9. In recent months several universities around the country have concluded multi-million dollar campaigns from private gift support constituencies. One has been completed at $350 million and another at $300 million. At least one medical school within the university's total achieved $150 million. During that same time, several universities have announced the launching of campaigns, with one as high as $1 billion. Often the medical schools' campaigns have goals of from $100 million to $250 million. These experiences would seem to indicate that the potential for private philanthropy is greater than it has ever been before and that, at least in comparison to the past experience, in capital campaigns the new goal figures are quite substantial.

10. The ——— School of Medicine believes that, despite the growth in private philanthropic support it has experienced over the past several years, the potential for private support of biomedical research is, at best, modest. While private support (including corporations, large and small foundations, individuals, and voluntary health organizations) to the School increased 10.5 percent from FY 1983 to FY 1985, this growth did not match the government research grants and contracts, which grew 17.5 percent.

A major drawback to private support is that such grants generally do not fully reimburse for indirect costs. As a result, there are costs to the institution in accepting private grants and contracts. As long as this policy remains in effect, institutions must carefully consider the impact of growth in private support for biomedical research.

These replies on the whole support the idea that private foundations and gifts from individuals hold promise of substantially enlarging the funding for biomedical R & D. However, this optimistic assessment does not mean that any of the AHC leaders anticipates that private philanthropy will be able to replace the federal government as the primary source of support for biomedical research.

Two further observations: None of the respondents referred to large-scale grants or contracts from industry. And several noted that, because of a small or nonexistent allowance for indirect costs, foundation and individual donations can add to the financial problems of a hard-pressed institution.

Question 2

Do such funds, to the extent that you have received them, provide more flexibility than governmental grants?

Replies

1. Funding from the private sector gives a great deal more flexibility than funding from a governmental agency because many donors are interested in a broad area of research, whereas federal support is usually for a specific project within a specific area of research.

2. Private funds provide far more flexibility than governmental grants. The most obvious example is our annual fund. It provides the Chancellor and our deans with funds which can be spent on research, teaching, or patient care. The federal government makes very few, if any, such unrestricted grants. The application and reporting process for private grants is far less cumbersome also.

3. In general, funds from foundations tend to be much more flexible than government grants. On the other hand they do not provide the support of overhead . . . We tend to lose three dollars in overhead recovery from governmental sources for every dollar lost in overhead for nongovernmental sources.

4. Funds from private sources have, in our experience, been less restricted in their use than comparable grants from federal sources. However, this is by no means always the case. As you know, some private donors have very narrow opinions about the uses to which they would like to see their money put. The procedures of private foundations regarding the allocation of indirect costs is a case in point.

5. The answer is emphatically yes to the flexibility question. You simply cannot get $2.5 million from the federal government to use as endowment to fund promising investigators and research in studies of pain, as an example.

6. With respect to flexibility, grants from major foundations have become at least as, and often even more restrictive than, those from the government with respect to the conditions attached. However,

the foundations are apt to refuse to pay overhead, so their grants can be viewed as more of a liability than an asset or assist.

7. Of course, private grants provide more flexibility than governmental grants, in terms both of use of funds and of reporting and accounting regulations.

8. Private funding does promise greater flexibility for medical schools. Because there is often an opportunity before funding to discuss with the donor (or foundation board) our specific circumstances, grant dollars can often be channeled more effectively than federal funds. Even in the case of restricted gifts, individuals usually are eager to assist the institution rather than to accomplish a narrow research objective.

9. In general, both the types of expenditures allowed in the use of private funds, i.e., capital and operating, and the minimal reporting required make these funds much more flexible than government grants. When the institution has an opportunity to work carefully with major donors, there is often more flexibility than funds from government support [allow]. Even though the funds may be directed toward a specific kind of research, there are usually fewer restrictions on the use of the funds in that process.

10. Foundation dollars are much more flexible than government dollars and are often more quickly acquired than government grants. It is possible to attract foundation dollars to develop new and innovative programmatic ventures for which government funding is not available. For example, the School of Medicine used a foundation grant to establish its internationally recognized Clinical Epidemiology Program. Three major private foundations provided the majority of the Program's initial funding and continue to do so. The flexibility of private dollars is integral to mounting new initiatives.

On balance, foundation and private donor support for biomedical R & D is viewed by the respondents as providing more flexibility than does governmental support. Specific attention is directed to less onerous reporting requirements, the ability to work with the donor in shaping the terms of the gift, and the speed of eliciting support when time is an important consideration. However, the disinclination of private donors to pay overhead or adequate overhead is repeatedly emphasized.

Question 3

Have potential donors or their lawyers or consultants explored such gifts before making them? Has your institution sought to engage the support of lawyers involved in trusts and estates to steer potential benefactors in your direction? Do you think such an effort would be worthwhile?

Replies

1. Most donors from the private sector discuss making a contribution, and how that contribution will be used, with members of the Board and Administration. We often, but only at the request of the donor, are in touch with lawyers involved in trusts and estates to provide information and to respond to questions. We do not seek out lawyers or consultants involved in trusts and estates to steer potential donors to our institution.

2. I strongly believe that an effort to involve lawyers and other financial advisors in the solicitation of private support pays off. To that end, we have an estate planning attorney working full time in the Development Office as the Director of Planned Giving. We have a Trusts, Annuities, and Bequests volunteer committee that includes advisors from various areas of expertise. This group has sponsored campus briefing luncheons for attorneys and CPAs and this fall will host a financial planning seminar for our alumni and friends. My Director of Planned Giving has informed me that she receives from one to three calls a week from attorneys requesting assistance in the wording of bequests, as well as information on other planned gift mechanisms.

3. Potential donors and lawyers have explored gifts before making them. We always welcome such interactions. I have often stated that our law school alumni are perhaps more important for fund raising than our medical school alumni. We do have a special program for interested lawyers regarding trusts and estates. It is a formal program presented once or twice a year in the ——— Center. It definitely pays off.

4. We do use consultants and lawyers in attempting to guide potential donors toward projects of interest to the School. Making contact with trust lawyers who have ——— Medical School in mind is not always easy. I would welcome increasing the size of the cadre of such individuals who are associated with our cause.

5. The answer to the third question is yes, and it does pay off handsomely.

Few donors, by the way, will give to totally unrestricted purposes. That, however, makes little difference since a gift for cancer research, as an example, usually helps free up other institutional resources for new uses.

6. Yes, it is rare for a significant gift to be made solely on the basis of a patient's gratitude to an institution or physician. However, the stronger the relationship with a doctor or institution, the more flexible and accepting of the institution's advice the donor is apt to be.

Yes, we do [engage the support of lawyers involved in trusts and estates to steer potential benefactors in our direction]. However, one must exercise great care so as not to give the lawyer or trust officer any sense that he is straying from the strict ethical standards of his profession.

7. We have not engaged consultants to solicit research support for us. Nor have we systematically asked lawyers involved in trusts and estates to steer donors in the direction of funding for research. Nevertheless, when the opportunity presents itself—for example, from time to time lawyers ask us for guidance in identifying funding opportunities for their clients—we recommend support for one of the two components of our current capital campaign: endowment for our medical school (which includes the endowment of research centers, research professorships and other research efforts) and support toward the rebuilding of the ——— Hospital. The same is true of potential donors: we try to steer them toward the support of institution-wide priorities, the most important of which is support for our Campaign.

8. In the case of major individual donors, we usually have advance contact with the donor or the donor's advisors to negotiate any restrictions included in the gift. The major exceptions are bequests. Often we are unaware of the donor's intent until probate. Even so, such final gifts often have broadly defined objectives, and we can work with executors to direct the funds most effectively.

9. It is becoming more and more common for donors and their attorneys or CPAs to work closely with the institution in the process of development of a major gift in order for them to realize the greatest tax benefits and for the institution to realize the greatest flexibility and potential value from the major gifts that are made. Attorneys and CPAs are becoming more aware and more sophisticated about the process and the need for it, and often suggest to clients that philanthropy be included in all estate and other financial planning. Major universities around the country have for a period of almost 20

years been doing a more thorough job of working with attorneys and financial consultants, and it has begun to pay off rather significantly.

10. On occasion, private foundations have established their own program foci and requested proposals within those guidelines. Individual donors have explored opportunities to establish and support new programs (e.g., disease-targeted research). The School of Medicine has not sought to engage the support of lawyers to steer gifts toward the institution, other than by using the legal services of the development office (these efforts, however, have not been to initiate such benefaction). The School has not yet developed a model to assess the degree to which such efforts might be successful.

These replies indicate that the responding AHCs differ significantly in their approaches to seeking out significant gifts. Some work closely with lawyers, accountants, other professionals, and supporters who might be helpful in identifying potential donors. Others follow a more conservative approach. Even the latter, once they are approached, seek to work closely with potential benefactors and their advisers in order to maximize the benefits of each gift to both the donor and the institution. Clearly, most AHCs are moving to strengthen their fund-raising activities.

Additional Comments of Respondents

In addition to the replies to the three questions, several of the respondents made comments about other aspects of the broad subject of philanthropic giving in support of biomedical research.

1. My feeling is that private foundations should provide the highest multiplier funds. My priorities have always been the support of:

   a. key people
   b. programs that emanate from key people
   c. physical facilities needed by these people.

2. One particular issue might be appropriate for your study. It is the great reluctance of private foundations to make grants for endowments. As you know, the development of a solid base of endowment for the support of independent research is essential for any private university or research institute. The style of operations of the private foundation in this country generally does not permit grants for such purposes. This means that virtually all endowment must come from private individuals. It would be very helpful if the attitude of the private foundation on this matter were to change. I am not hopeful, but perhaps a review of this problem in your report could work in the direction of improving the situation.

3. Quite simply, I think what is happening is the consolidation, within a relatively few institutions, of the major national research effort. Those that have the critical mass of researchers and the ability to make resources available, together with private funding for start-up costs, are simply going to garner more and more research funding from both the NIH and private sources.

4. Your study of private philanthropic support of biomedical research is timely. As the impact of the federal budget deficit becomes more clear, pressures will mount to trim medical research expenditures. Few options exist to replace that support, and the capacity of private philanthropy to do so has not been fully explored.

The prospects for private philanthropy are substantial, but the future is clouded by several major uncertainties. Will shareholders continue to endorse the growing presence of corporations in the charitable arena? To what extent will the entry of public universities and small non-profits into that arena dilute the charitable dollar? How will tax reform alter the ways in which individual Americans support medical schools?

In spite of my reservations, I remain optimistic that our private support will grow rapidly. By making greater efforts to reach our constituencies, we can persuade them that their help is crucial to a healthier society, something of great interest to the American people. The philanthropic urge is deep-seated in the American ethic, and medical research can claim an even larger share of attention, if medical schools do a better job of explaining their role in the nation's health care system. I see your project as one step in that process.

In their additional comments, the respondents reaffirmed their belief in the considerable potential of private philanthropy as a source of financing for biomedical R & D at the same time that they expressed some uncertainty about the impacts of the new tax legislation. On balance, they came down on the optimistic side.

Two other points were stressed: the importance of funds for endowments and the possibility that in a period of funding stringency biomedical research will increasingly be concentrated in the limited number of strong institutions that have the requisite funds to survive and prosper.

Teaching Hospitals

To round out the survey, the authors requested the most recent annual reports and financial statements of thirty large teaching hospitals that were not the principal affiliates of medical schools. Our aim was to assess the extent to which philanthropic entities, particularly private foundations and individual donors, were making sizable gifts to these institutions. In 1985 the NIH awarded $150 million in grants to hospitals not intimately connected with institutions of higher education. Clearly, some large independent teaching hospitals are engaged in biomedical research.

Of the thirty large teaching hospitals, only fourteen submitted usable information. Several informed us that they do not routinely publish annual reports, and some failed to include financial data in sufficient detail to enable us to assess the role of philanthropy in supporting biomedical research at their institutions.

There was one outlier among the fourteen hospitals from which we received pertinent material. This hospital had annual philanthropic receipts of $55.5 million in 1985, up from $38.2 million in 1983. Four hospitals received gifts of between $6 and $11 million; two received $3.5 million and $2.2 million respectively; four received funds in the $1–2 million range; and the remaining two received $270,000 and $140,000 respectively.

After reading the annual reports and analyzing the accompanying financial statements, we concluded that the five recipients of the largest philanthropic gifts are substantially or moderately engaged in biomedical research; however, research was not a significant activity in the remaining hospitals.

A number of generalizations and inferences can be drawn from the analysis of the experience of this group of major research-oriented AHCs that bear on the role of philanthropy, particularly private foundations and individual donors.

—Although the proportion of federal funding for biomedical research has declined over the years, the federal government remains by far the principal source of research support of the major AHCs.

—It would be a reasonable inference that, during the years when federal grant money was increasing rapidly, investigators concentrated their efforts on the NIH and other government agencies since these were the most favorable sources from which to seek funding for their research. Their relative neglect of philanthropic sources reinforced the tendency of foundation trustees and staff to cede the responsibility for the funding of basic biomedical research largely to the federal government.

—In the decade of the early 1970s to the early 1980s, when federal dollars for biomedical research became more difficult to obtain, the AHCs came to realize that they had to explore alternative funding sources, and some have moved a considerable distance toward focusing more of their fund-raising efforts on existing and potential philanthropic sources.

7 · The Potential for Philanthropy

The point has been made many times that, with a preference for small government, Americans have resorted to philanthropy to finance many socially valuable objectives. In point of fact, no advanced country has expanded its philanthropic giving as much as the United States. As we noted earlier, the total of such giving in 1986 came to $87 billion, with the health area the recipient of about $12 billion or 14 percent.[1]

Although philanthropy played a leading role as a provider of biomedical research funds in the pre–World War II era, and thereafter in constant dollars its contributions grew fivefold, the dominant role after World War II that the federal government assumed in financing biomedical research led to a striking relative decline in philanthropy's share of the total.[2]

This chapter explores the potential of philanthropy to become a more important source of funds for biomedical research in the years ahead, a challenge that gains importance in the face of continuing pressures on the federal budget. Such an exploration requires examination of both the macro forces affecting potential total giving and giving for health and the micro fund-raising outlook of the major medical research centers.

The Macro Outlook

The most striking potential macro development is the goal that the Independent Sector has set for total giving in 1991. The objective is to raise from voluntary sources $160 billion, or approximately double the amount collected in 1985. If this target is achieved or approximated, and if the health arena is able to maintain its current share of circa 14 percent, it would receive over $22 billion. The present contribution to biomedical research of $700 million annually from all philanthropic sources (see table 2.2), about 5 percent of total health giving, would in turn be about half again as high as its current level, or roughly $1.1 billion. If the philanthropic share of health funding for biomedical research increased from 5 percent to just above 6 percent and the ambitious goals for total giving were realized, philanthropy's support of biomedical research would approximately double, reaching a level of around $1.4 billion in 1991.

In the light of recent trends in giving and in the medium-term outlook for the economy, it is problematic, however, that the Independent Sector's goal will be realized by 1991. Since the end of the recession in 1982, the subsequent period of economic growth and lowered inflation produced a 45 percent increase in total giving from $60 to $87 billion.

Unless one postulates that the United States and the rest of the world are about to enter upon a period of sustained growth, it is difficult to anticipate that total giving will more than double its recent rate of growth. The Organization for Economic Cooperation and Development, the International Monetary Fund, and the World Bank were of one voice in 1987 in pointing out that the U.S., West European, and Japanese economies are falling short of their optimal levels.[3] Many analysts believe that they will continue to fall short unless they can individually and jointly effect the following developments: a reduction in the U.S. government deficit and trade imbalance; reduced volatility in exchange rates; a restructuring of Third World debt; and the avoidance both of protectionism and of the renewal of inflation. Though the level of philanthropic giving is likely to continue to rise in the absence of a severe and prolonged recession—and possibly even in the face of such an untoward event—caution suggests that the five-year goal of doubling contributions is not likely to be realized and that maintaining even the recent rate of growth will be a creditable achievement.

If one looks at two of the four component sources of giving, foundations and corporations, which together accounted for just over $9.7 billion, or 11 percent of all giving in 1986, it is difficult to imagine that their grant policies will be altered to such an extent that their contributions will become significantly more important in the funding of biomedical research. They, together with the rest of society, may respond to the growing AIDS crisis by making additional grants for basic or applied research, but it is unlikely that such crisis actions will have a significant impact on their total level of support for biomedical research. It is important to note that even those foundations that view health as their principal area of concern, such as the Robert Wood Johnson Foundation, the Commonwealth Fund and the Henry J. Kaiser Family Foundation, have not made significant grants for biomedical research in recent years.

There are two notable exceptions, the Howard Hughes Medical Institute, which with $5 billion in assets is the world's largest philanthropy, and the Lucille P. Markey Charitable Trust.[4] The Hughes program is currently carried out by 33 research laboratories in academic medical centers, hospitals, and universities located throughout the United States, with 178 investigators and approximately 1,400 employees in the scientific program. Biomedical research is conducted in five broad areas: cell biology and regulation, genetics, immunology, neuroscience, and structural biology. The total budget of $230 million in 1988 is scheduled to rise to $242 million by next year. With the initiation of a new grants program, an additional $500 million will be spent over the next ten years to support education in the medical and biological sciences.

The Howard Hughes Medical Institute is a medical research organization, (MRO), not a private foundation. However, through a stipulation by the IRS, Hughes may nevertheless fund outside research once it expends 3.5 percent of its endowment on internal research.

The Markey Charitable Trust awarded grants amounting to $75.4 million in 1987, an increase of $33.7 from 1986. Since the corpus of the estate has been conservatively estimated at $300 million and possibly considerably more if the price of oil recovers, and since all of the trust's assets must be paid out by 1997, it is clear that Markey, although much smaller than Hughes, is currently and potentially a significant funding source for biomedical research.

A smaller but significant funder of biomedical research has

emerged from the reorganization of the James S. McDonnell Foundation. In 1986 its total health-related awards came to over $4 million, and in 1987 the sum had risen to $4.6 million, almost all of which was devoted exclusively to the support of biomedical research.[5] Finally, the Josiah Macy, Jr. Foundation, a relatively small philanthropy, spent $2.6 million in support of 13 grants at 10 institutions in the area of pathobiology between 1981 and 1986.

We will now look more closely at recent grant-making decisions of the major foundations, particularly those with a past or present interest in health, in order to assess whether and to what extent they currently support biomedical research or are likely to do so in the near term.

The Rockefeller Foundation, which historically has played a leading role in supporting biomedical research in this country and abroad, in 1985 allocated $5.7 million, or 11.3 percent of its total grants, for "health sciences," up from $4.2 million, or 9 percent of the total, in 1983.[6] Supporting the claim that "the overall aim of the Health Sciences program is to improve the health of mankind, with a particular emphasis on the developing world," its 1985 report notes that the foundation funds biomedical research to develop new and better drugs and vaccines, trains clinical epidemiologists to develop cost-effective means of disease treatment and control, and devotes funds to disseminating biomedical and health information. Its network of fourteen units working on the "great neglected diseases of mankind"—malaria, schistosomiasis, hookworm, and recurrent diarrheas in children—is distributed among many different lands, although several of the clinical laboratories are in the United States.

The Ford Foundation in 1986 approved programs that totaled $180 million in six major fields.[7] Health has not been a designated area of the Ford Foundation's support, except in relation to its ongoing interest in population problems. Included is the effort to improve "the quality and effectiveness of family planning and reproductive health programs," with a heavy emphasis on programs in the Third World.

The Andrew W. Mellon Foundation has long been interested in supporting programs aimed at reducing population pressures, particularly in the Third World.[8] Between 1977 and 1985 the foundation made grants totaling more than $50 million for these programs, including support for research projects in reproductive biology.

Seven pages of grants categorized as for medicine, public health, and population and totaling just under $17 million dollars are listed in the 1985 report of the Mellon Foundation. Included are three-year grants to fifteen major private medical schools, amounting to $5,350,000, which "will make possible . . . continued junior faculty appointments for a number of able young scientists to carry them through immediate post-doctoral years to a point at which they are eligible for tenured teaching appointments or can compete independently for research support."[9]

Although the Alfred P. Sloan Foundation noted in its annual report that "the costs of research in the mainstream of science and engineering . . . have moved well beyond our financial range and have become the responsibility of government, industry and research institutions themselves," it made a large $2.5 million one-time grant in 1985 to the Sloan-Kettering Institute for Cancer Research for research in molecular biology and virology, cell biology and genetics and immunology. Other grants were awarded for molecular studies in evolution, research fellowships in neuroscience, and work in computational neuroscience. The total of these exceeded $4 million, a considerable sum, in view of the foundation's earlier avoidance of the financing of research, including biomedical research.[10]

In recent years the Pew Memorial Trust has become a significant supporter of biomedical research.[11] Starting at an annual level of about $4.5 million during the years 1979–83, the Pew Trust group allocated $16.9, $21.4, and $10.9 million respectively for the years 1984–86. In addition, sizable related grants for the support of medical education and hospital construction and renovation were awarded.[12]

The John A. Hartford Foundation inaugurated a fellowship program in 1979 to promote the career development of young physicians interested in pursuing medical research.[13] It provided three-year grants to twelve fellows every year with a stipend of $45,000. Because of the trustees' conviction that ample alternative sources for such funding had become available since 1979, they decided in 1985 to terminate the program. Currently the foundation has two major program interests: the Health Care Cost and Quality Program and the Aging and Health Program. Biomedical research is no longer a focus of its support.

The John D. and Catherine T. MacArthur Foundation directed $11 million of its $63.5 million total allocation in 1985 to health. It has made "substantial, ongoing commitments to the major world health problems—mental health and parasitic diseases." Unlike most foundations, MacArthur directs resources "primarily to research programs generated and developed by Foundation staff and advisors . . . Its strategies include encouraging interdisciplinary collaboration . . . and supporting the next generation of investigators."[14]

The Robert Wood Johnson Foundation, one of the largest foundations in the world with annual grants of about $90 million, is devoted exclusively to the arena of health.[15] Since the foundation began its grant making on a national basis in 1972, it has distributed approximately $750 million. At no time during the 1970s or following its reassessment of program objectives in the early 1980s has biomedical research been an area of primary or even secondary concern. The foundation's objectives have been to improve access to health care for individual groups, make health care more effective and affordable, and help people maintain or regain maximum function. In the twenty-one pages of grants authorized in the year ending 21 December 1986, as detailed in its 1986 report, only a few can be found that are even tangentially related to biomedical research. In its 1988 reassessment of its program objectives, the foundation has again excluded biomedical research as a target area.

There are three other foundations with long-established interests in health: the Duke Endowment, the Commonwealth Fund, and the Henry J. Kaiser Family Foundation.[16] Each has much more modest resources than the Johnson Foundation, and they have for the most part eschewed allocating any significant part of their annual disbursements for biomedical research. In 1985 the Duke Endowment awarded about $14 million for health, primarily for hospitals and other health care delivery systems in North and South Carolina, the area that defines its geographical scope of operations.

A major program initiative of the Commonwealth Fund, which in 1986 disbursed $4.4 million in health grants, was directed to "strengthening academic health centers"; the project subsequently received over one-fifth of the fund's allocations. One of the principal aims of this effort was to identify ways of strengthening the infrastructure of the AHCs, including their capacity to continue effective work in biomedical research.

In 1985 the Kaiser Family Foundation made just over $9 million available for health-related programs and projects. About two-thirds of these grants were for education and training. Recently the foundation has decided to focus attention on community-based prevention and health promotion programs aimed at reducing morbidity and mortality growing out of dysfunctional life styles.

The W. K. Kellogg Foundation directed 36 percent of its funding in 1985–86 to health, which was its primary area of investment.[17] The foundation, which has been operating for fifty-six years, had expenditures in excess of $80 million in 1986, placing it among the largest philanthropic organizations. The 1986 report notes that "the Foundation seldom funds basic or laboratory research." Most of its program activities could best be described as action-based or applied research. In the early 1980s the foundation identified its interest in the health arena as "betterment of health through health prevention and public health, and community-wide, coordinated, cost-effective health services."

In sum, giving by foundations interested in health may be summarized as follows:

—Johnson, the largest of the health-focused foundations, has had no direct interest in biomedical research since it initiated its broad grant program in 1972.

—Several large foundations such as Mellon and Sloan have made and continue to make significant contributions to the training of young researchers and to selected program areas of biomedical research.

—By far the two largest funders of biomedical research among the foundations are Hughes and Markey.

—Pew, MacArthur, and McDonnell are significant new players in the biomedical research arena.

—Some of the smaller health-focused foundations such as Hartford, Duke, Commonwealth, and Kaiser are not currently making any significant grants for biomedical research.

The Micro Outlook

Another vantage point from which to assess the potential of philanthropy for biomedical research is to focus on the fund-raising activities of selected large private universities and medical research institutions to gauge their recent efforts and success in raising philanthropic funds.

In his financial report for the year 1986, Michael Sovern, president of Columbia University called attention to certain dimensions of the university's fund-raising activities that bear directly or indirectly on biomedical research.[18] He noted that during the course of the year the university had received gifts totaling $94.5 million, of which $46.3 million came from alumni and other individuals. This sum indicates the importance of individual giving to a major research-oriented university. Sovern noted that, by the end of 1986, the university had passed the 82 percent mark in its goal of raising $500 million. At the close of the campaign in 1987, total gifts had exceeded $600 million.

Specifically, he described the fund raising for the university's Health Sciences Campus.

The Columbia Presbyterian Medical Center officially kicked off a $245 million fund-raising campaign and began the largest hospital construction and modernization program in the world. Donations are being used to expand and renovate existing hospital facilities, construct a new 745-bed hospital at the Medical Center, endow 28 senior professorships and 29 junior faculty posts in the health sciences, provide more student aid . . . By year's end the CPMC Fund was approaching $140 million . . . Improvements at the Health Sciences campus planned for 1986–1987 include additional work on our animal care facilities as well as renovation and modernization of laboratories for the Biochemistry, Cellular Biophysics, Medicine, Microbiology, Obstetrics and Gynecology, Orthopedic Surgery, Physiology, and Urology Departments.[19]

Since 1980 the university had spent about $95 million on deferred maintenance throughout the Morningside and Health Sciences campuses, had issued $130 million in new tax-exempt bonds to help finance future capital programs, and had participated in a pooled state offering that would eventually provide an additional $22 million to finance the purchase of equipment.

These efforts call attention to the critical roles that two aspects of philanthropy continue to play: that of gifts in providing funds for the maintenance and improvement of the capital plant and equipment; and that of contributions to the endowment in helping to cover the salaries of key faculty members and in providing flexibility in meeting other operating expenses. Only those universities and medical schools that have adequate capital plant and equipment in place to pursue both basic and clinical research projects and, in addition, command sizable endowment funds to help cover the salaries of research investigators are in a position to compete successfully for government grants for biomedical research.

The Supporting Schedule for the medical school, the College of Physicians and Surgeons, attached to Sovern's financial report provides additional information about the role of philanthropy in the operation of a major research-oriented institution.[20] It reveals that the medical school has 39 distinct financial subunits, exclusive of the Nursing School, the School of Public Health, and the School of Oral and Dental Surgery, all of which are administratively independent of the medical school. The total expenditures for the College of Physicians and Surgeons in 1986 for "instruction, research, and educational administration" came to $194.8 million. If the $30.7 million expended for the operation of Harlem Hospital, a New York City hospital affiliated with Columbia, is subtracted, the core outlays of the medical school came to $164.1 million. The following departments, institutes, centers, and divisions each had expenditures in excess of $5 million: Anesthesiology, Population and Family Health, Health Sciences, Medicine, Neurology, Obstetrics and Gynecology, Pathology, Pediatrics, Psychiatry, Radiology, and Surgery.

Expenditures from government grants and contracts amounted to $82.6 million in 1986, just about one-half of the school's total outlays. The medical school recovered $29.3 million for indirect costs, which means that out of a total of $111.9 million received from the government for R & D, the investigators had slightly less than three out of four government R & D dollars to spend on their direct research.

The Supporting Schedule showed that investment income for the College of Physicians and Surgeons came to just under $8 million and that private gifts, grants, and contracts amounted to $16.1 million.

Included in this last sum are awards from industrial foundations and industry of $5.3 million. In addition, endowment and gift income of $2.1 million was recorded under the heading "Medical School Administration." In short, as far as operating income is concerned, philanthropy, supplemented by industrial foundations and awards, contributed over $24 million to the funds under the direct control of the medical school, or to its budget of $164 million (excluding Harlem Hospital). In addition, the university, as we noted earlier, expended over $46 million on plant and equipment, some part of which redounded to the advantage of the Health Sciences Campus.

When the current campaign for the medical center has been completed, the new endowment funds for senior and junior faculty will represent a further annual philanthropic contribution of the order of $3.5 million.

This long exegesis on the flow of funds for the support of one large research-oriented medical school was presented in order to provide a base for questioning the macro finding that philanthropy contributes only about 3–4 percent to total funds for biomedical research. The figures that were culled from the financial report of Columbia University for 1986 suggest that the total share of philanthropy at major research centers is considerably larger, in this case five times larger in fact, than the reported national average.

In order to determine whether the figures for Columbia University, particularly its medical school, are representative of major research-oriented institutions, we compared them with figures for New York University and the University of Pennsylvania, which have been among the top 20 institutions in terms of NIH funding during the past eighteen years. The spring 1987 issue of *NYU Physician* entitled *NYU Salutes the NIH* contains a breakdown of the NYU Fund's support for the New York University Medical Center for the period 1 September 1985 to 31 August 1986.[21] The center had a restricted budget of $87.4 million. Of this total, the federal government, primarily the NIH, contributed 69 percent; state and local government, 1 percent; business and industry, 3 percent; foundations and private health organizations, 7 percent; gifts, endowments, and all other sources, 20 percent. If the last two categories are combined, philanthropy accounted for $23.5 million, or about 27 percent.

In connection with the ceremonies marking the dedication of

the Founders' Pavilion at the University of Pennsylvania Medical Center in September 1987, a construction effort amounting to $96 million, information about the financing of the medical center's operations over the last decade was made available. In fiscal year 1986 investment and gift income amounted to $14.8 million, and nonfederal grants and contracts amounted to another $10.2 million, for a combined total of $25 million, or 12.1 percent, of total revenue of $206.6 million.

It becomes increasingly clear that the presumption that philanthropy contributes between 3 and 4 percent of all funding for biomedical research is questionable. This low figure fails to reflect much of the investment income from endowments and philanthropic funds raised for capital and equipment. Were it not for these sizable contributions, it is unlikely, once the federal research dollars began to slow, that the AHCs would have been able to maintain their key roles as the largest performers of biomedical research and the dominant performers of basic research.

It should be observed that the broadening of the categories of philanthropic support for biomedical research to include funds for capital plant and endowment is not fully congruent with the flow of federal funding for biomedical research, which no longer includes more than small amounts for such purposes.

The question that remains is the potential of institutions of higher education, and particularly their medical centers, to increase the flow of gifts from individuals and bequests. In pursuing this line of inquiry, we will look more closely at some of the key points that emerged in the replies of the medical directors to our questionnaire, reported in chapter 6.

Although some of the respondents were concerned about the potential impact of tax reform on philanthropic giving, experience since passage of the tax reform act of 1986 suggests that most of these fears were exaggerated.

More importantly, the respondents emphasized that they, and others in leading positions at AHCs, realized that they had neglected to cultivate potential donors, particularly the new millionaires, but believed that once they mounted a focused and sustained effort, the results would be positive. In fact, they pointed to recent gains in fund raising, gains that in their opinion could be increased substantially once they put an efficient fund-raising structure in place with interested volunteers and competent staff.

Though the primary spur to enlarged philanthropic fund raising for AHCs stems from the new interest and concern of the deans and faculty members, note must also be taken of the initiative of the occasional large private foundation whose founder or trustees have decided to single out biomedical research as the area of their special concern.

One of the largest foundations with a special interest in funding biomedical research has defined its strategy thus: Recognizing the impossibility of providing a major offset to declining federal funds, the foundation singled out a critical area for support, one in which investigators from different disciplines are working at the frontiers of science and results are attainable only in the long term. Accordingly, the foundation has identified universities and medical schools with strong faculty who are currently working on the frontiers of biomedical research in an area such as developmental biology. The foundation realizes that if prestigious research groups are supported for a number of years during which they can pursue new approaches and develop new techniques, they will be in a better position to compete for sustaining grants from the federal government. Hence it sees as its challenge and responsibility the funding of high-risk, high-return work through the early stages of exploration and discovery. In pursuing this strategy, the foundation has returned to the classic role of philanthropy, the provision of seed money for basic research, a role that many foundation have lost sight of as a consequence of their preoccupation with the here and now. The dynamics of contemporary science underscore the need for more venture capital for basic research.

Midway in the campaign to raise $450 million for Johns Hopkins University by 1990, the School of Medicine and the hospital had received $185.7 million in gifts and pledges by May 1987. Included in the list of "10 specific goals to be accomplished during the remaining part of the campaign," were "unrestricted funds for the Hospital and Medical School, research buildings, endowed chairs for senior faculty, clinical-scientist funds." Clearly, philanthropy was being asked to do more, much more, for biomedical research.

The Hopkins campaign card is indicative of the broadened efforts that the fund raisers are making to interest potential contributors.

The summer 1987 edition of *Hopkins Medical News* included a

THE CAMPAIGN FOR JOHNS HOPKINS

Many alumni/alumnae and friends have already included Johns Hopkins in their financial plans. If you have done so, or would like information on the various options and their benefits, we would like to know. Please check as many boxes as you like.

- ☐ *I have included Johns Hopkins in my will, trust, or other financial plans.*
- ☐ *I would like information on the tax and income benefits of gifts of:*
  - ☐ *appreciated securities* ☐ *real estate* ☐ *life insurance* ☐ *antiques, artwork, etc.*
- ☐ *I would like to know more about gifts which provide:*
  - ☐ *income to me for my lifetime* ☐ *income to Johns Hopkins and assets to my heirs*
- ☐ *I would like specific legal language to include Johns Hopkins in my will.*
- ☐ *Please call me at* ____-________; *best time to call is* ________

Name ________________

Address ________________

City ________________ State ________ Zip ________

short article entitled "Bequests Promote Hopkins Vitality."[22] In 1986 the school of medicine and the hospital received more than $4.4 million from the estates of twenty six alumni and friends. Three gifts of $1 million or more were for "faculty support." Six of twelve in the amount of $100,000–999,999 explicitly mentioned research, and several others were for endowment, faculty support, or unrestricted purposes. Included in the remaining eleven bequests of up to $100,000 were four exclusively for research and several others for endowment, faculty support, or unrestricted purposes.

There are other signs that point to an expanded role for philanthropy in the funding of biomedical research. The Dana-Farber Cancer Institute in Boston, the origins of which date back to 1947, had not sought to develop a significant endowment until the Dana Foundation made a challenge grant to the institute of $10 million in 1982. The institute had to match the first $5 million of the grant and had to raise $15 million to qualify for the second $5 million of foundation funding. During the period of the challenge, the institute increased its endowment from $1.5 million to more than $43 million and increased the overall goal of its first major capital campaign to $50 million.

On a related front the National Multiple Sclerosis Society took the initiative in December 1986 to explore with representatives of large medical foundations, academic leaders, and senior officials of the NIH the question "Should the hard-won dollars of single-disease-oriented voluntary agencies be spent on patient services or on lobbying to obtain a larger NIH budget, rather than on research?"[23] The participants at the meeting reached consensus on several issues including:

—The society should not stop supporting research.
—A solid program of grants and fellowships must remain the centerpiece of any meaningful research program.
—An important part of the society's research budget should be assigned to pilot research, that is, the testing of new ideas.
—New types of training support are needed to promote recruiting MDs into research.
—Imaginative new programs of biomedical research are needed that emphasize cooperation (bridging).
—The society should not direct a major part of its research into lobbying or increasing public awareness of multiple sclerosis.

While the national health agencies have long appreciated the importance of educational efforts aimed at increasing the level of their donations and further using their enlarged membership to help persuade Congress to increase its research funding for expanded efforts to conquer specific diseases, industry for the most part has attended to its own knitting and has not sought allies among the philanthropic community.

Recently Pfizer, in one of its health care series, has stressed that medical research—"building a healthier future"—stems from a partnership that includes the NIH, universities and teaching hospitals, and private industry laboratories. The message emphasizes that medical research is an expensive process and that "we must all do our part to help keep the flow of discoveries active and ongoing." It provides the following answers to the question, What can you do? "*Speak up*: Let your legislators know that you want funding of biomedical research by NIH and other federal government agencies to be kept at the highest possible levels. *Contribute* to voluntary health organizations supporting disease research."[24]

For the first time since the federal government became the principal funder of biomedical research after World War II, industry is making an effort to inform the American people of the interconnections among the key partners, government, academia, philanthropy, and itself.

But there is nothing easy in forging and maintaining an effective alliance among the critical parties that in the final analysis shape the level of congressional support for biomedical research: the NIH leadership, the guardians of the budget in the Executive Office, the congressional leadership, and the interested constituents on the outside, particularly the members of the research community.

The director of the NIH recently recalled how the NIH lost funding and later the authority to fund extramural construction. He emphasized that "we saw no particular response from the extramural community." A similar lack of response from the research community resulted in the recent loss of grant programs for the support of institutional research. The administration had sought repeatedly to delete these funds, but Congress had reinstated them. "This year that hasn't happened." As a concerned congressman said to the NIH director, "The extramural community really let you down this year."[25]

8 · Open Issues on the Nation's Biomedical Research Agenda

In conclusion, we will flag some of the more important issues on the nation's biomedical research agenda, some of long standing, others recent. These issues have attracted the attention of the major centers of power such as the Congress, the academic community, business leaders, the public, and the press.

The following selected macro issues have recently attracted attention:

—Washington, the press, and the business community are increasingly concerned about the loss of competitiveness of the U.S. economy and the threat of further erosion. While the explanations have focused on a host of factors, from ineffective managerial leadership to contentious labor-management relationships, another line of analysis stresses the greater investments that the leading countries of the Organization for Economic Cooperation and Development (Germany, France, the United Kingdom) and Japan are directing to civilian R & D.[1] Although the United States devotes approximately the same proportion of its GNP to R & D as do its major competitors, circa 3 percent, two additional points should be noted. First, a disproportionate share of U.S. expenditures is directed to defense and defense-related activities. Though these activities have spillover effects on the civilian sector (commercial aircraft, computers, communications equipment), their impact is likely to be less than if the R & D were directly focused on civilian and commercial goals. Second, the possible imbalance between the defense and civilian sectors of the R & D effort has heightened significance if the premise is accepted that the most promising growth center for high-tech economies is about to shift from computers, which are entering their fifth decade, to biotechnology, which is just taking off.

—In 1986 a challenging article was published in the *New England Journal of Medicine* under the title "Progress against Cancer?" which concluded that, despite the substantial and continuing large-scale federal and other expenditures on research directed to understanding the causes of and seeking the cures for cancer, overall incidence and prevalance rates, with the exception of a limited number of uncommon forms of the disease, have remained level or have increased, and survival rates have not improved over the last several decades.[2] Although the findings led to acrimonious rebuttals by senior officials of the National Cancer Institute and by members of the research community who read the evidence differently, many sectors of the press and the public concluded that the initial promise of the NIH to use federal funds to find cures for many diseases involved a far more complex and extended process than many of the proponents of large federal support had appreciated or acknowledged.

—This tension between the level of research funding and the lag in finding cures for the targeted diseases has recently surfaced in the federal government's response to the AIDS epidemic. Many believe insufficient leadership and resources, particularly resources for research, have been brought to bear on the problem. In early 1988, Congress is finally, with the administration's acquiescence if not enthusiastic support, planning to appropriate $1 billion for AIDS research and education. Up to this time both the executive and Congress have dragged their feet when it came to responding to the growing crisis. For some time the administration's policy was to avoid the issue, then to deflect some NIH funds to AIDS research, and later possibly to reappropriate a part of Medicare's large budget to fund a limited number of AIDS proposals.

—During the recent past, several major research universities, facing serious shortages of space and equipment, have engaged influential lobbyists in Washington in an effort to obtain congressional support for certain of their high-priority projects. Several universities were successful in persuading key members of Congress to add their projects to appropriations bills without the usual process of peer review. Many journalists have referred to this process as pork barrel legislation. Cornell University, which was awarded $10 million through such special legislative largesse, decided that it would not accept the award.[3]

This list provides a highly selective introduction to the large number of policy issues bearing on R & D in general and biomedical research in particular that are on the nation's agenda. This chapter focuses on selected issues that relate specifically to the future role and vitality of biomedical research within the context of the earlier analysis, which emphasized the potential for the contributions of philanthropy. We will consider sequentially several open issues that relate to the levels of future financing, to the universities' and medical schools' infrastructures, and to changing relationships among the key parties—the federal government, academia, industry, and the public.

Future Financing

We noted in chapter 5 that there is no single indicator or even multiple indicators that can provide reliable guidance about how much a nation such as the United States should spend on biomedical research. The best reference points appear to be: the path of past spending; the expenditures of other advanced nations; the rate of growth of the nation's GNP, including in particular the condition of the federal budget in light of the importance of federal support for basic research.

The 1988 presidential budget, which contains forecasts through 1992, recommends that "total spending for the Public Health Service remain capped." Most of the reduction of $10.7 billion over the next five years is to be "achieved through limiting research funding for the National Institutes of Health."[4] However, the president's proposal may well be just that, a proposal rather than a guideline or a certainty.

—Capping the expenditures of the NIH would reverse the trend of the recent past (since 1982–83), during which additional federal funds were appropriated for biomedical research after a decade of only desultory increases in the levels of federal support.

—With rare exceptions, Congress has repeatedly increased the successive administrations' budgetary proposals for the NIH. Upward revisions have also been characteristic of the Reagan administration. A reasonable presumption is that Congress will not accept the president's capping proposal. To illustrate: In 1978, 1979, and 1980 the congressional appropriations for the NIH were approximately $300 million above the president's budget. Beginning in 1984 the gap between budget and appropriations has widened to between $400 and $600 million.

—Three factors may lead the legislators to increase the future level of funding for the NIH. The first is the unsatisfactory state of the universities' research facilities; the second, the relatively low percentage of approved NIH grant proposals that are currently being funded; the third, the upward drift in the average expenditure per researcher per annum.

On the question of facilities the former long-term chairman of the House Science and Technology Committee, Don Fuqua, who headed a science policy study before his retirement in 1986, concluded that "our universities are basically strong, healthy, and appreciated, but they have drifted into a critical situation involving the research infrastructure. Some immediate direct action must be initiated . . . Ten billion dollars, half of which would come from matching money, would do much to alleviate the situation."[5] Fuqua added that unless new money becomes available, the rebuilding of infrastructure should be paid for by curtailing grant support for individual researchers.

The Panel on the Health of U.S. Colleges and Universities (the Packard-Bromley Panel) of the White House Science Council, reporting in 1986, also singled out facilities and equipment as requiring early replacement action if U.S. research universities are to be in a position to respond to the multiple demands that American society continues to make on them.[6] The members of the panel believed that the additional funding recommended should come in considerable measure through a reallocation of R & D appropriations from applied research and development to basic research, but they also emphasized that incremental new funding would be required.

The Packard-Bromley Panel also called attention to the unrealistic criteria that the federal government has used to reimburse universities for the depreciation of facilities and equipment and recommended radical changes in the guidelines for depreciation, including assuming a useful life of twenty rather than fifty years and, in the case of equipment, five to ten years, rather than fifteen. The panel warned, however, that if these recommendations are followed, indirect costs should not draw money from direct research but should come from a reallocation of funds from other sources. The panel explicitly disagreed with Representative Fuqua's recommendation that new funding for facilities be covered in part by reducing the support for research grants by an order of 10 percent.

Both the panel and Fuqua favored a 50 percent matching requirement from institutions, states, and private sources. The panel put the matter thus: "State and local governments as well as private philanthropy, play a vital role. Their initial investments develop the structures and programs that make universities competitive for federal investment, and they provide the resources by which academic institutions preserve their automony and diversity. Moreover, such support is a major element of the shared responsibility that typifies the present university–federal government partnership."[7]

Several points are worth attention. Without support for buildings and equipment, the major research universities will not be able to compete effectively for federal R & D funds. While the primary emphasis of the Packard-Bromley Panel's report was on the university–federal government partnership, it also recommended avenues through which industry could increase its role by supporting continuing educational programs at universities for its scientific and engineering personnel and for the federal government to establish problem-oriented research centers directed to meeting broad national needs and to furthering industrial technology.

Included in the sixty-two recommendations of the report of Representative Fuqua, which is still to be released in its entirety, are some that relate specifically to biomedical research:

I believe there is little likelihood that the pace of medical research will be permitted to slacken because the results have been too impressive and too gratifying to permit a loss of momentum in this area. The populace as a whole will demand the rapid-paced continuation of medical research, and the Congress for the most part will provide the means for its accomplishment.

Our present progress would seem to indicate that we are devoting a reasonable and responsible portion of our tax dollars to health research. Any large increase in funding would not likely lead to a commensurate spurt of accomplishment because break-through researchers are limited in number, most are adequately funded already, and there is time required for maturation of ideas. More effort should be made, however, to discontinue support of marginally productive researchers and in the process make certain that young investigators get a chance to launch their careers.[8]

There is one more federal initiative that bears on the future structure and financing of biomedical research. The National Science Foundation has sought appropriations to fund a number of basic science and technology centers in the belief that such centers could have several beneficial effects: they would stimulate interdisciplinary research at the frontiers, facilitating collaboration among biologists, chemists, and chemical engineers in a biotechnology center; they would make it easier for industrial researchers to interact with basic scientists, and as a result technological breakthroughs could be speeded and the competitiveness of the U.S. economy could be enhanced.

In his 1987 state of the union message, the president called attention to a new initiative: the establishment by federal agencies of science and technology centers. He described these as "new university-based interdisciplinary 'Science and Technology Centers' that will focus on fundamental science that directly contributes to the nation's economic competitiveness." The National Science Foundation has elicited proposals with the aim of funding some of these new centers in the near future.

In February 1987, Erich Bloch, the director of the National Science Foundation and a principal advocate of these centers, sought guidance from the National Academy of Sciences. The academy established a panel, which held two meetings and issued a report that emphasized its views on principles and guidelines.[9]

In its final chapter, entitled "Some Cautionary Observations," the report warned about the diversion of funds from grants to individual investigators and cautioned strongly against a repetition of the situation involving the Defense Department's University Research Institute, which, because of lack of new funding, weakened the existing basic research programs of the military services.

The panel issued other warnings, including the possibility of excessive competition for resources; the risk that centers might become unresponsive to new ideas and unreceptive to new people; the necessity for cross-disciplinary research of national resources; the danger that the objective of accelerating the transfer of technology could lead to a narrow focus on near-term commercial applications; and the possibility of reducing healthy competition in a relatively small scientific field by the establishment of one or two centers.

Problems that the new centers would not solve were also noted: insufficient funds, support of too short duration, obsolete equipment, and inadequate staffing. But the panel's final conclusion was that the proposed new centers could make significant contributions to science and the nation's economic competitiveness if they could have proper management, resources, and evaluation and if the National Science Foundation would maintain a healthy balance among the principal modes of research support.

The development of science and technology centers is not restricted to federal initiatives. The states of North Carolina and Pennsylvania undertook some years ago to invest in infrastructure that encouraged the concentrated location of science-based industries in the "Research Triangle" in the Chapel Hill–Raleigh–Durham area and in the Philadelphia area respectively.

A current illustration of such public-private cooperation is the recently signed agreement among the State of New York, the City of New York, and Columbia University for the funding and construction of "the first university-industry research building in New York City dedicated to commercial development of biomedical technology." The proposal provides for the construction of a four-story, $22 million building with a floor area of 100,000 square feet adjacent to the Columbia-Presbyterian Medical Center. Forty percent of the building will be reserved for start-up companies. The university will be the developer of the project, invest $4 million as equity, and manage and operate the facility. The city will invest $10 million and the state $8 million, to be repaid by the university. The state's congressional delegates assisted in launching the project by modifying the 1986 tax reform act to allow favorable financing for the program.[10]

Another variant was the $3 million start-up contribution of the John A. Hartford Foundation in 1985 to the University of Texas Health Science Center at Dallas "to facilitate more effective commercial application of its biomedical research through an innovative agreement with the Dallas Biomedical Corporation. The newly-formed corporation will invest in promising projects, using interest from $12 million provided by local investors. The Foundation's grant will match funds from the Corporation on a project-by-project basis."[11]

What guidance can be derived from this review of selected forces that are likely to have an impact on the future financing of biomedical research?

—The unbalanced federal budget and the likelihood that balance will not be achieved within the next five years emphasize the barriers to any significant increase in the level of funding of biomedical research by the federal government, which has been and remains the principal sponsor of basic research.

—The Reagan administration's concern with present and prospective budgetary deficits has led it to recommend capping the NIH budget for the next five years, that is, through 1992.

—In the opinion of the Congressional Budget Office, such recommendations with respect to the NIH are not likely to be accepted by the Congress.[12]

—Both the Packard-Bromley Panel and former Representative Fuqua called attention to the need for early action to modernize the research infrastructure, both buildings and equipment. Representative Fuqua estimated that such an effort across all R & D activities at university campuses would require an investment program of about $10 billion, half of which should be funded by the federal government, and half by state and local governments and philanthropy. The Packard-Bromley Panel looked to a reallocation of federal R & D expenditures and some additional federal financing to cover the federal government's share; Fuqua was willing to shift some grant support funds to the urgent task of modernizing the research infrastructure.

—The administration has been pursuing a policy of allocating more federal support to basic research, and it has reaffirmed this stance in supporting more funding for the National Science

Foundation, part of which is to finance new centers for science and technology.

—It was Representative Fuqua's opinion that Congress would continue to support biomedical research liberally but that there was little prospect of large-scale congressional increases in the current level of support. He recognized the need to free up grant support money for young investigators and recommended that this be accomplished by reducing and eliminating support for investigators who were only marginally productive.

—The Packard-Bromley Panel, recognizing the conflict between its desire to see more funds flow to academia, primarily for strengthening basic research, and the importance of not adding to the federal deficit, looked to some reallocations from the $100 billion expended nationally for R & D to increase the flow of funds to the research universities.

Brief note should also be taken of two related areas that have affected and are likely further to affect the relationships between the federal government and the universities in the funding of basic research. The first concerns the recent rise in real costs of the support required to keep one full-time investigator productively employed in research and teaching students. The other has been the intensified friction between government and the universities over the unresolved issue of overhead costs, specifically the amount of universities' overhead that the federal government should cover in its research grants.

A recent report by the Division of Policy Research and Analysis of the National Science Foundation (February 1987) presented data that indicate a basic stability in constant (1984) dollars in the average cost of a full-time employee–year at universities and colleges, which amounted to $140,000 during the extended period 1966–81. In the last five years the figure has increased to $155,000, and the report estimates that it is likely to reach $180,000–205,000 by 1997.[13]

The report emphasizes that this rise in the amount needed to support a full-time employee will require an input of an additional $7 billion in constant dollars by 1996 or a cumulative inflow to universities and colleges of $30 to $40 billion from all sources over the decade. It adds that these figures are the minimum required to maintain the present level of academic R & D and do not reflect the additional dollars that would be needed if the nation decides to fund some large projects, increase the number and quality of graduate students and researchers, or engage in more technologically focused research. Reformulated, these figures suggest that the flow of federal and other dollars into universities will have to be significantly increased if the nation is to maintain its current level of basic research in the several sciences, including biomedical research.

Once external funds for research became a significant part of the annual revenues of major research institutions, it was inevitable that these institutions would become more aware of the full costs to them of space, administration, library and related technical services, maintenance, and security, which are affected by the size of their externally funded research activities. Greater sophistication in their internal cost accounting systems permitted more accurate estimates of specific costs, and this in turn led the institutions to intensify their efforts to recapture these costs in subsequent negotiations with the federal government. The Office of Management and Budget has done its best to keep the universities' claims for additional overhead from undue escalation. In the effort at containment it has steadily promulgated more rules and regulations; until recently, universities had to report the percentage of time that faculty members spent on their research as distinct from other duties, such as teaching or patient care.[14]

We noted in chapter 2 the marked increase in the proportion of total grant money that overhead costs claim. The issue of upward creep in indirect costs has been the cause of considerable tension among academic administrators, researchers, and federal officials. The efforts of the research universities to extract from the federal government an ever-larger amount for overhead reflects in large measure the unwillingness of the federal government to make any general fund support available to them.

Two recent developments warrant attention. When the Packard-Bromley Panel recommended that the revision of Circular A-21 of the Office of Management and Budget set a limit on overhead costs, it was a step in the right direction. The panel suggested that the costs be fixed at a "uniform percentage of modified total direct costs of the research . . . based on the mean national percentage over a five-year historical period" to be phased in over a two-year period. After heated discussions with the representatives of academia, the proposed circular was revised to cap departmental administrative costs as one way of capping total indirect costs. The panel's recommendation that investigators no longer be required to report the amount of their time and effort spent on research was accepted.[15]

The long-term arguments between the Office of Management and Budget and the major research universities over allowable overhead on research grants has not been settled. At best the capping of departmental administrative costs has provided some short- and middle-term relief to the federal government, which is understandably concerned that more and more of its project money is not being made available to research investigators for their current expenditures but is being preempted to cover institutional overhead.

At the instance of Senator Lawton Chiles, chairman of the Senate Budget Committee, studies were initiated, first in Florida and then in other parts of the country, to address the broad question of the burden of unnecessary federal administrative regulations imposed upon the research universities and their faculty members.

The head of the Policy Office of the National Science Foundation had been moving his agency toward the concept of block grants without administrative controls and without accountability for funds but with accountability for research accomplishment. Several major universities including the University of California, Columbia, Florida State University, the University of Florida, Johns Hopkins, the University of Miami, the State University of New York, and the University of Virginia agreed to participate in the new collaborative effort at administrative simplification of grant procedures.

The findings of the case studies carried out at Columbia University involving such matters as the costs entailed in the preparation of noncompeting proposals, foreign travel approval, equipment approval, preparation of reports of expenditures, and six other administrative requirements indicated that "at least $100 million could be saved at research colleges and universities throughout the country if these ten federal administrative requirements were eliminated."[16]

The elimination of faculty time-and-effort reporting, the reduction in the number of items that universities had to keep under administrative surveillance and report to the federal government, the movement toward block grants that would permit the research investigator to comingle funds from multiple sources, and the emphasis on evaluating the progress made toward the stated research goals—all are clearly moves in the direction of freeing up investigators' time.

Further, if the federal government, in an era of constrained dollars, is to obtain a reasonable amount of research effort for its outlays, the overhead costs claimed by the research institutions and universities must be capped.

There are unquestionably many additional reforms that joint efforts between the research universities and the Office of Management and Budget could identify and implement if they succeed in reestablishing mutual trust. It would be unrealistic, however, to expect that with an annual flow of federal funds amounting to between $50 million and $500 million per major research institution, paper work could be largely eliminated. The important point is that the most important capital of research investigators is their time, and increasingly elaborate administrative controls inevitably reduce their productivity.

There is another difficulty that the AHCs face in a period in which cross-subsidization in their major teaching hospitals is being severely restricted as a result of tightening reimbursement practices by third-party payers. The principal academic centers have long engaged in varying amounts of unfunded clinical research. The costs involved were included in patient bills. But the new emphasis on competitive pricing makes it increasingly difficult for a large teaching hospital to write off these unfunded research costs through surcharges on patients' bills. A recent estimate indicates that in a large research hospital such unfunded research costs might add about $110 per discharge, no great amount when compared to a typical bill of $5,000 or more, but still sufficient to add strain to an institution that is facing a declining patient census and a smaller margin.[17] The concentration of most unfunded clinical research in a relatively few institutions underscores that, though the problem is limited in scope, finding a solution is important to the major centers that carry out most of the clinical research.

The aim of the preceding discussion is to call attention to the perspectives and trends that are likely to bound the financing of biomedical research in the closing decade of this century.

—The key funder, particularly for basic research, is likely to remain the federal government. No other sector, neither industry nor philanthropy, has the interest or the resources to replace the federal government, which today covers about 90 percent of the total expenditures for basic biomedical research.

—The strained circumstances of the federal government's budget and the modest efforts that have made in recent years to bring it back into balance make it unlikely that the federal government will be able to increase or possibly even to maintain the upward trend in its outlays for biomedical research that has characterized the last five years.

—The pressures for continued increases, however, are considerable: the threat of a national AIDS epidemic; the growing recognition that additional investments must be made in the research infrastructure if future research productivity is not to be undermined; the steeply rising costs of equipment and support for full-time researchers; the growing belief that the United States must make special efforts to protect and strengthen its technological lead in order to protect its international competitiveness, which includes biomedical research and biotechnology.

—Some developments are underway, and more may be just over the horizon, that point to some moderation of demands on the federal government to cover as much of the total biomedical research bill as in years past. A growing number of states have come to appreciate the importance of investing in research and technology as a preferred way of enhancing their economic development and per capita income. As we noted in chapter 7, universities, and particularly ACHs, have become much more aggressive in fund-raising activities including the identification of new potential donors who have recently acquired substantial fortunes. Finally, industry has recognized that synergistic gains are possible from closer ties, financial and other, between itself and the major research universities, which remain the principal performers of biomedical research.

A conservative estimate would see the federal government as

continuing to be the predominant funder of biomedical research at century's end. But it is likely that the share contributed by state governments, industry, and philanthropy will also increase and that together these three sources will account for considerably more than one-half of all funding for biomedical research and perhaps up to one-quarter of the funding for basic research.

Interactions among the Key Parties

Thus far this chapter has focused on policy issues involving the continuing role of the federal government in the financing of biomedical research. Now it is both necessary and desirable to consider at least briefly the other principal parties—particularly the research universities and medical schools, philanthropy, and industry—in terms of their areas of activity and their interactions with one another.

As we have shown, there is a growing consensus among informed observers that the research infrastructure of higher education needs to be refurbished and both Fuqua's committee and the Packard-Bromley Panel expect the universities to obtain matching funds from philanthropy and from state and local government. With the total estimated backlog of construction and equipment for all R & D estimated at $10 billion, the 50 percent share of biomedical research funds to be raised from philanthropy and the states should not prove overly burdensome.

The point made by the Packard-Bromley Panel is worth reemphasizing: research universities with a strong infrastructure of buildings and research staff already in place are in a preferred position to compete effectively for federal biomedical research funds. Without both, they will lose out. It is therefore essential that the progress they have begun to make in intensifying their fund-raising efforts from alumni, friends, foundations, and bequests—reviewed in the preceding chapters—be pursued and intensified. Philanthropic dollars have substantial leverage.

The universities, particularly the AHCs, face several new challenges that may complicate their research mission in the years ahead.[18] We noted earlier that the single largest source of medical school revenue, particularly for the major private research-oriented institutions, is income from practice plans. This means that an increasing proportion of the clinical faculty must see paying patients in order to help earn their salaries and contribute to the expenses of running their departments and the medical school itself. But seeing and treating patients reduces the time they have for research and teaching.

Another complication arises from the planned reduction of reimbursement by Medicare for large teaching hospitals engaged in graduate medical education. The federal government is covering the training costs for residents only up to first certification (three to five years). This means that the AHCs must find alternative sources to cover the training of specialists and subspecialists who are essential if clinical research is to flourish.

Shifting our focus from the research institutions to philanthropy, we find that the total annual contributions of philanthropy to health are considerable—in excess of $12 billion, a sum equal to three-quarters of the national total of $16 billion for all biomedical research. But of this sizable philanthropic total, by far the smallest proportion—in the 3–4 percent range—is specifically directed to biomedical research. A considerable sum goes for patient care services, and the largest amount goes for construction. Some part of the latter, of course, contributes to strengthening the infrastructure for biomedical research.

However, our earlier analysis pointed to the possibility in the quinquennium ahead of substantial increase in philanthropic giving for health that, as we have pointed out, may lead to a doubling of total donations. If such an increase were to materialize, the current and prospective needs of the research institutions for more capital and operating funds for biomedical research would be easier to cover. But it is clear that philanthropy has not yet recognized biomedical research as a major area of importance. The two most hopeful developments are the anticipated expenditures of the Howard Hughes Institute of at least $300 million annually and the potential that the medical leadership believes exists to tap other sources, particularly new wealth, once prospective donors have been identified and cultivated.

This brings us to a brief consideration of the role of industry in the future financing of biomedical research. We noted in earlier chapters that industry has been expanding its absolute and relative shares of financing for biomedical research to a point where it accounts today for more than two out of every five dollars. However, these dollars are primarily for applied research and development, not for basic research, and a growing proportion of industry's annual spending for biomedical research takes place outside the United States.

At the beginning of this decade, a number of large chemical and pharmaceutical companies, U.S. and foreign, made large grants for basic research to a limited number of major U.S. research universities and AHCs. The donors sought to strengthen their positions in what appeared to be the coming breakthrough in biotechnology. The arrangements that they worked out with the universities and other research institutions gave them first call to exploit the discoveries that resulted from their largesse.

The intervening years have led to some reassessment by both academia and the corporate sector. As the survey reported in *Science* in early 1986 by David Blumenthal and his associates emphasized, though many biotechnology companies continue to make grants, they are generally at modest levels and for short durations.[19] The mega-grants of the early 1980s have not been repeated. One reason appears to be that the role of process engineering is viewed as increasingly critical in transforming the new knowledge gained in the laboratory into new products in the marketplace. To the extent that this continues to be the case, large companies will find it increasingly desirable to internalize their development work. The growing linkages between small venture capital biotechnology firms and multinational pharmaceutical and chemical companies, as well as buy-outs of the former by the latter, point in the same direction—the need for a strong corporate infrastructure to transform a new idea into a new product.

Consequently it is unlikely that industry will become a major source of funds for basic research in biotechnology at the nation's academic research centers. Further, academia has encountered difficulties in adjusting to external funding sources that are interested in developing proprietary products. To mention a few that Blumenthal and his coauthors noted: the deflection of academic talent to second-order problems that may yield profits to the funder; the inhibitions of faculty members about discussing their work freely because they do not want to reveal proprietary information; restrictions on publication; and still other types of behavior that are not in the academic tradition of the free exchange of ideas.

Blumenthal and his associates believe that corporate funding for university research in biotechnology contains too many benefits to be rejected outright, but he made a plea to the universities to consider how they can continue to benefit from such funds without placing their basic values at risk.

Among the more interesting issues that have appeared on the agenda of science policy is the question of whether large-scale funding should be provided to enable biologists, with the assistance of other scientists, to map and sequence the entire human genome. As the spring 1987 number of *Issues in Science and Technology* made clear, there are strong supporters and opponents of the transformation of biology into big science on the particle physics model.[20] While everybody agrees that the major mapping-sequencing effort would prove valuable for future investigations, the opponents point to the costs of accomplishing the task, given the relatively large amounts of capital and scientific talent required to carry out the effort in the face of the still embryonic technology available for sequencing.[21]

George F. Cahill, Jr. of the Howard Hughes Medical Institute has pointed out that neither side has "placed sufficient emphasis on the greatest problem in mapping and sequencing: the handling, storage, and most important, the interpretation of the data."[22] The NIH estimates that it currently spends about $300 million to support some three thousand research projects related to the elucidation of complex genomes, both human and nonhuman. Of this sum about $90 million is for studies directly related to the human genome.

It is highly unlikely that the United States will assume its share of the calculated cost of $6 billion to sequence the entire human genome at the present time, especially since technological breakthroughs might, within a decade or so, cut the cost to $60 million.

As of 1988 it is by no means clear when the long-anticipated breakthrough in biotechnology will occur or what the further rate of the industry's expansion will be once the breakthrough has occurred. There is still good reason to believe that continuing advances in biomedical research and the development of biotechnology hold promise of important new processes and products that will contribute to the improved competitiveness of the U.S. economy. But the overriding reason for broad-scale national support of biomedical research remains today, as was stated in the Bush report of 1945, the advancement of knowledge and improvement in the health of the American people.

The focus of this analysis has been on the critical role of financing in sustaining a desirable level of national effort in biomedical research. Our analysis called attention to the following problem areas:

—The inability of the NIH, even under recently expanded appropriations, to support more than two out of every five proposals that are judged worthy of being funded.
—The need for more capital investments in facilities and for the purchase of new equipment and instrumentation.
—The increasing difficulties that the major AHCs face in continuing to charge patients for the costs entailed in unfunded clinical research.
—The likelihood that the initial reduction in Medicare reimbursement for graduate medical education will place in jeopardy the training of an adequate number of qualified specialists and subspecialists in clinical research.
—The growing perception among leaders of the medical establishment, as well as federal and state legislators, of an emerging surplus of physicians and the desirability of reducing the capacity of medical schools, which carries with it the likelihood of reduced financing for both medical education and biomedical research.
—The financing dilemma posed by the fact that the federal government has long been and remains the principal funder (financing about 90 percent) of basic biomedical research, as well as the funder of much of the infrastructure, and the severe budgetary constraints that confront the federal government at present, which are not likely to be removed in the near term. This predicament calls for larger efforts by the other funders—industry, state government, and philanthropy. And, as the Packard-Bromley Panel suggested, it also calls for a future reallocation of existing federal funding from applied research and development to basic research.
—In a special report for the Office of Technology Assessment, Louis Harris and Associates undertook in the fall of 1986 a

national probability sample of American adults to elicit their views about science, technology, and genetic engineering, including their views about funding for biological research.[23] Though 43 percent of respondents, the largest group, favored a continuation of the present level of funding and 10 percent thought the level should be cut "somewhat" or "substantially," 39 percent favored higher levels of funding. The remaining 7 percent "didn't know." Support for enlarged expenditures was bipartisan, although Democrats were slightly more favorable to larger outlays than Republicans. There were only minor differences among adults with varying levels of education: 40 percent of high school dropouts and 45 percent of college graduates favored larger expenditures.

Critical as adequate funding is to assure the vitality of the biomedical enterprise, even more critical is the attraction of talent from the nation's pool of human resources. The number of young people of high potential who are interested in pursuing a research career in biomedicine is relatively limited, and biomedicine faces severe competition from other high-prestige domains—the professions, finance, management, public affairs, and above all, other scientific disciplines.

The United State faces a series of unfavorable population trends in the years ahead, that is, up to the end of this century. First and foremost, the nation is in a demographic dip: the number of twenty-year-olds is declining from around 4.3 million in 1983 to about 3.4 million in the year 2000, or by roughly one-fifth. These totals mask the fact that in the years ahead, blacks and Hispanics will represent a growing proportion of the young adult population. Since these minorities are grossly underrepresented among those who attend college and graduate school, the effective pool for biomedical research personnel is further constrained. In addition, the teaching of mathematics and science in the nation's secondary schools has been found to be seriously deficient by a number of distinguished commissions and committees, a condition that does not lend itself to easy or speedy correction. A further complication has been the distortions introduced by the booming financial markets of recent years, which have been able to attract, because of the prospects of high initial earnings, disproportionate numbers of talented college graduates, including those with a strong science background.

On the positive side, we noted earlier that a number of foundations have recognized the strategic importance of supporting talented young investigators during the formative years of their careers to the point where they can compete successfully for NIH grants and for a tenured position in an AHC. Further, several foundations are also making funds available to encourage talented young physicians to broaden and deepen their research training in the hope that some of them may decide to become career investigators.

While the financing of biomedical research must seek to meet the needs of established investigators, it must at the same time assure that adequate funds are available to maintain tomorrow's talent pool. The promise of biogenetics and biotechnology has never been greater. But the realization of that promise depends on creating the educational opportunities and the career positions that will attract and retain a sufficiently large number of able young people to advance the frontiers of science, to contribute to the expansion of biotechnology, and to increase the preventive and curative powers of medicine.

Notes

Chapter 1. Overview

1. U.S. Department of Health and Human Services, National Institutes of Health, *NIH Data Book*, 1987 (Bethesda, Md., December 1987). The figure for 1940 is from the NIH Office of Program Planning.
2. Ibid.
3. U.S. Congress, House, Science and Technology Committee, Science Policy Study, Don Fuqua, chairman, *Recommendations* (Washington, D.C.: Council on Government Relations, 11 November 1986); U.S. Executive Office of the President, Office of Science and Technology, White House Science Council, Panel on the Health of U.S. Colleges and Universities, *A Renewed Partnership* (Washington, D.C., February 1986).
4. U.S. General Accounting Office, *University Funding. Information on the Role of Peer Review at NSF and NIH*, GAO-RCED-87-87FS (Washington, D.C., March 1987).
5. Erich Bloch, "Basic Research and Economic Health: The Coming Challenge," *Science*, 2 May 1986, 595–99; National Academy of Sciences, *Science and Technology Centers: Principles and Guidelines* (Washington, D.C., 1987).

Chapter 2. The Funding and Performance of Biomedical Research and Development

1. Eli Ginzberg and Anna B. Dutka, *The Financing of Biomedical Research in the United States, 1950–1985. A Chartbook and Text* (Conservation of Human Resources, Columbia University, March 1986), Mimeograph; U.S. Department of Health and Human Services, National Institutes of Health, *NIH Data Book* (1987). Data for 1940 are from the NIH Office of Program Planning.
2. Vannevar Bush, director of the Office of Scientific Research and Development, *Science: The Endless Frontier. A Report to the President on a Program for Postwar Scientific Research* (Washington, D.C.: USGPO, July 1945).
3. *Science*, 21 August 1987, 847.
4. Stephen L. Strickland, *Politics, Science and Dread Disease* (Cambridge: Harvard University Press, 1972).

5. James A. Shannon, "The National Institutes of Health: Some Critical Years, 1955–1957," *Science*, 21 August 1987, 868.

6. U.S. Department of Health and Human Services, National Institutes of Health. *Biennial Report of the Director*, vol. 1, 1985–86, DHHS, NIH Pub. no. 87-2912, June 1987.

7. Victoria A. Harden, *Inventing the NIH: Federal Biomedical Research Policy, 1887–1937* (Baltimore: Johns Hopkins University Press, 1986), 186.

8. *NIH Data Book*, 1987, table 31.

9. David Blumenthal, Michael Gluck, Karen S. Louis, and David Wise, "Industrial Support of University Research in Biotechnology," *Science*, 17 January 1986, 242–46; David Blumenthal, Michael Gluck, Karen S. Louis, Michael A. Stoto, and David Wise, "University-Industry Relationships in Biotechnology: Implications for the University," *Science*, 13 June 1986, 1361–72.

10. Gerard F. Anderson and Catherine M. Russe, "Biomedical Research and Technology Development," *Health Affairs*, Summer 1987, 85–92.

Chapter 3. Investment in Biomedical Research: Critical Ratios

1. Vannevar Bush, director of the Office of Scientific Research and Development, *Science: The Endless Frontier. A Report to the President on a Program for Postwar Scientific Research* (Washington, D.C.: USGPO, July 1945), vii.

2. Ibid., 1, 11.

3. Eli Ginzberg and Anna B. Dutka, *The Financing of Biomedical Research in the United States, 1950–1985. A Chartbook and Text* (Conservation of Human Resources, Columbia University, March 1986), mimeograph; 1987 data added.

4. National Science Board, *Science Indicators: The 1985 Report*, NSB-85-1 (Washington, D.C., 1987), appendix table 2–12; U.S. Department of Health and Human Services, National Institutes of Health, *NIH Data Book*, 1987 (Bethesda, Md., December 1987).

5. National Science Board, *Science and Engineering Indicators: 1987*, appendix table 4–5; National Institutes of Health, *NIH Data Books* (Bethesda, Md.).

6. National Science Board, *Science and Engineering Indicators:* 1987, appendix tables 4–6, 4–18.

7. U.S. Congress, Congressional Budget Office, *An Analysis of the President's Budgetary Proposals for Fiscal Year 1988* (Washington, D.C., February 1987).

8. Ibid., 112.

9. Ibid., 111.

10. John P. Swann, *Academic Scientists and the Pharmaceutical Industry* (Baltimore: Johns Hopkins University Press, 1988), 170–71.

11. U.S. Congress, House, Committee on Ways and Means, Subcommittee on Health, testimony by Robert F. Allnutt, 2 June 1987.

12. Penny Peace and Howard Berliner, "The Changing Structure of the Pharmaceutical Industry," report to U.S. Congress, Office of Technology Assessment, June 1985, mimeograph; Pharmaceutical Manufacturers Association, *U.S. Trade in Drugs and Medicinal Chemicals: Analysis of Trends and Forecasts to 1990* (Washington, D.C., June 1987).

13. Pharmaceutical Manufacturers Association, *1987 Annual Report* (Washington, D.C., 1987).

14. Michael R. Pollard and Gary S. Persinger, "Investment in Health Care Innovation," *Health Affairs*, Summer 1987, 100.
15. *Financial Times*, 1 October 1987, sections III, I.
16. Peace and Berliner, "Pharmaceutical Industry," 32–33.
17. Pollard and Persinger, "Investments," 99–100.
18. Peace and Berliner, "Pharmaceutical Industry," appendix table 15.

Chapter 4. How Many Dollars Are Enough?

1. Vannevar Bush, director of the Office of Scientific Research and Development, *Science: The Endless Frontier. A Report to the President on a Program for Postwar Scientific Research* (Washington, D.C.: USGPO, July 1945), 8. Emphasis in original.
2. Ibid.
3. Julius H. Comroe, Jr. and Robert D. Dripps, *The Top Ten Clinical Advances in Cardiovascular-Pulmonary Medicine and Surgery 1945–1975*, final report, DHEW Pub. no. (NIH) 78-1521, 31 January 1977, 3, 89.
4. Robert W. Berliner and Thomas J. Kennedy, "National Expenditures for Biomedical Research," *Journal of Medical Education* 45 (September 1970): 666–78.
5. Ibid., 675.
6. Ibid., 676.
7. Ibid., 677.
8. Selma J. Mushkin, *Biomedical Research: Costs and Benefits* (Cambridge, Mass.: Ballinger, 1979).
9. Ibid., 9.
10. National Academy of Sciences, National Academy of Engineering, Institute of Medicine, Committee on Science, Engineering, and Public Policy, *The Federal Role in Research and Development*, report of a workshop (Washington, D.C.: National Academy Press, 1986), viii, vii.
11. Ibid., 6–7.
12. Ibid., 10.
13. Ibid., 17.
14. Ibid., 18.
15. Zvi Griliches, "R & D and Productivity: Measurement Issues and Economic Results," *Science*, 3 July 1987, 31–35.
16. Bush, *Science: The Endless Frontier*, 50.
17. Ibid., 58.
18. Ibid., 53.
19. Ibid., 41.
20. Ibid., 58.
21. Louis Harris and Associates, *The Bristol-Myers Report: Medicine in the Next Century*, study no. 861018 (New York, 4 March 1987).

Chapter 5. The Philanthropic Dimension

1. American Association for Fund-Raising Counsel (AAFRC), Trust for Philanthropy, *Giving USA: Estimates of Philanthropic Giving in 1986 and the Trends They Show*, 32d annual issue (New York, 1987).
2. U.S. Department of Commerce, Bureau of the Census, *Statistical Abstract of the United States, 1987* (Washington, D.C., 1987).

3. Taft Group, *The Taft Corporate Giving Directory* (Washington, D.C., 1987).
4. Benjamin Lord, *Corporate Philanthropy in America: New Perspectives for the Eighties*, a Taft special report (Washington, D.C.: Taft Group, 1984), 7.
5. *New York Times*, 30 July 1987, letters to the editor.
6. AAFRC, *Giving USA, 1986*, 82–92.
7. Ibid., 83.
8. Zoe E. Boniface and Rebecca W. Rimel, *U.S. Funding for Biomedical Research*, a report prepared for the Pew Charitable Trusts (Philadelphia, April 1987).
9. Robert J. Blendon, "The Changing Role of Private Philanthropy in Health Affairs,"*New England Journal of Medicine*, 17 May 1975, 946–50.
10. Betty L. Dooley, *Health Giving Patterns of Philanthropic Foundations 1975, 1980, and 1983* (Washington, D.C.: Center for Health Policy Studies, Georgetown University School of Medicine, 1987).
11. Ibid., 17.
12. Boniface and Rimel, *U.S. Funding*, chapter 4.

Chapter 6. Academic Health Centers

1. Commonwealth Fund, *Prescription for Change*, report of the Task Force on Academic Health Centers (New York, 1985).
2. *Journal of the American Medical Association*, annual special issue on medical education and medical financing, 26 September 1986.

Chapter 7. The Potential for Philanthropy

1. American Association for Fund-Raising Counsel, Trust for Philanthropy, *Giving USA: Estimates of Philanthropic Giving in 1986 and the Trends They Show*, 32d annual issue (New York, 1987).
2. Eli Ginzberg and Anna B. Dutka, *The Financing of Biomedical Research in the United States, 1950–1985. A Charbook and Text*, (Conservation of Human Resources, Columbia University, March 1986), mimeograph.
3. International Monetary Fund, *World Economic Outlook*, April 1987 (Washington, D.C., 1987); World Bank, *World Development Report 1987* (New York: Oxford University Press, 1987).
4. Howard Hughes Medical Institute, *Grants Program of the Howard Hughes Medical Institute* (Bethesda, Md., 1987); Lucille P. Markey Charitable Trust, *Annual Report, 1986* (Miami, Fla., 1986).
5. Communication from James S. McDonnell Foundation, St. Louis, Mo.
6. *The Rockefeller Foundation, President's Review and Annual Report, 1985* (New York, 1986).
7. *Ford Foundation 1986 Annual Report* (New York, 1987).
8. *Report of the Andrew W. Mellon Foundation, 1985* (New York, 1986).
9. Ibid.
10. Alfred P. Sloan Foundation, *Report for 1985, Report for 1986* (New York, 1986, 1987).
11. Pew Memorial Trust, *Annual Report 1985* (Philadelphia, 1986).
12. Zoe E. Boniface and Rebecca W. Rimel, *U.S. Funding for Biomedical Research*, report prepared for the Pew Charitable Trusts (Philadelphia, April 1987).

13. John A. Hartford Foundation, *1985 Annual Report* (New York, 1986).
14. MacArthur Foundation, *Report on Activities*, 1985 (Chicago, 1986).
15. Robert Wood Johnson Foundation, *Annual Report*, 1986 (Princeton, N.J., 1987).
16. *The Duke Endowment, 1985* (Charlotte, N.C., 1986).
17. W. K. Kellogg Foundation *1986 Annual Report* (Battle Creek, Mich., 1987).
18. Columbia University, *Financial Report 1986* (New York, 1987).
19. Ibid., 6–7.
20. Supporting Schedules in ibid.
21. New York University School of Medicine, *NYU Physician*, Spring 1987.
22. Johns Hopkins Medical Institutions, *Hopkins Medical News* 11, no. 1 (Summer 1987).
23. Arthur K. Asbury, Clifford H. Goldsmith, and Byron H. Waksman, "The Role of Voluntary Agencies in the Funding of Biomedical Research," *New England Journal of Medicine*, 25 June 1987, 1665.
24. Pfizer, Inc., advertisement, *The Sciences*, May-June, 1986, 28–29.
25. *Science*, 21 August 1987, 842.

Chapter 8. Open Issues on the Nation's Biomedical Research Agenda

1. National Science Board, *Science Indicators: The 1985 Report*, NSB-85-1.
2. John C. Bailar III and Elaine M. Smith, "Progress against Cancer?" *New England Journal of Medicine*, 8 May 1986, 1226–32.
3. Cf. *New York Times*, 22 May 1987, "40 Universities Agree to Reject Disputed Grants."
4. U.S. Congress, Congressional Budget Office, *Reducing the Deficit: Spending and Revenue Options. 1987 Annual Report* (Washington, D.C., January 1987), and *An Analysis of the President's Budgetary Proposals for Fiscal Year 1988* (Washington, D.C., February 1987).
5. U.S. Congress, House, Science and Technology Committee, Science Policy Study, Don Fuqua, chairman, *Recommendations* (Washington, D.C.: Council on Government Relations, 11 November 1986), no. 4.
6. U.S. Executive Office of the President, Office of Science and Technology, White House Science Council, Panel on the Health of U.S. Colleges and Universities, *A Renewed Partnership* (Washington, D.C., February 1986).
7. Ibid., 4.
8. Fuqua, *Recommendations* no. 33.
9. National Academy of Sciences, *Science and Technology Centers. Principles and Guidelines*, a report by the Panel on Science and Technology Centers (Washington, D.C. 1987), viii.
10. *Columbia University Record* 13, no. 1 (17 July 1987).
11. John A. Hartford Foundation, *1985 Annual Report* (New York, 1986).
12. Congressional Budget Office, *Analysis*, iii.
13. National Science Foundation. *Future Costs of Research: The Next Decade for Academe*, PRA Rept. 87-1 (Washington, D.C., February 1987).
14. U.S. Executive Office of the President, Office of Management and Budget, *Circular No. A21—Revised Transmittal Memo. No. 2 and No. 3* (Washington, D.C., 4 and 9 June 1986).
15. Ibid.

16. Columbia University, Office of Projects and Grants, *OPG Newsletter*, vol. 9, 11 May 1987.

17. Gerard F. Anderson and Catherine M. Russe, "Biomedical Research and Technology Development," *Health Affairs*, Summer 1987, 85–92.

18. Eli Ginzberg, *American Medicine: The Power Shift*, (Totowa, N.J.: Rowman and Allanheld; 1985).

19. David Blumenthal, Michael Gluck, Karen S. Louis, Michael A. Stoto, and David Wise, "University-Industry Relationships in Biotechnology: Implications for the University," *Science*, 13 June 1986, 1361–72.

20. See the following articles in *Issues in Science and Technology*, Spring 1987: Walter Gilbert, "Genome Sequencing: Creating a New Biology for the Twenty-First Century," 26–35; Leroy Hood and Lloyd Smith, "Genome Sequencing: How to Proceed," 36–46; David Baltimore, "A Small Science Approach," 48–50; Francisco J. Ayala, "Two Frontiers of Human Biology: What the Sequence Won't Tell Us," 51–56.

21. "Forum: Genome Sequencing," special section of *Issues in Science and Technology*, Summer 1987.

22. George F. Cahill, Jr., Communication, "Forum: Genome Sequencing"; special section of *Issues in Science and Technology*, Summer 1987, 5.

23. Louis Harris and Associates, *Public Attitudes toward Science, Biotechnology and Genetic Engineering*, study no. 863012 (New York, 9 July 1987).

Index

The Financing of Biomedical Research

Designed by Ann Walston

Composed by BG Composition
in Trump text and display type

Printed by BookCrafters
on 50-lb. Booktext Natural text stock,
and bound in Holliston Roxite cloth